Jordan,

Thank you for y

kindness and encouragemen

and for your willingness

to read my book.

It means alot! :)

♡
Audrey

Klonopin Withdrawal
& Howling Dogs
Maybe it was God

Audrey Wagner

ISBN:0692291008
ISBN-13:9780692291009

The events in this story are true. The dialogue, timeline, and details are expressed as authentically as possible based on my fallible memory and, in the case of my childhood back story, by the recounting to me of some conversations I was not present for. Organization names and some personal names were changed, and city names were changed or fabricated. My book contains suicidal ideation and other potentially disturbing content. It contains Christian spirituality. My book does not provide or intend to serve as scientific or statistical information about withdrawal from Klonopin or any class of drugs. My book is not intended as medical advice or advice for whether or how to withdraw from any medication. I am not responsible for any decisions that any individual makes as a result of reading this book.

Audrey Wagner

PREFACE

Before I wrote this book, I studied how to write fiction so that I could tell my nonfiction story creatively. This guidance from other writers was indispensable. Yet for all I learned, I feel I lack the ability to fully capture the moment-to-moment suffering I experienced when discontinuing Klonopin. I believe my descriptions fall quite short, but I do hope they are sufficient to communicate my story.

CONTENTS

ACKNOWLEDGMENTS

I thank Ashleigh Siskar for reading my book in one of its close-to-final drafts. Her feedback was very encouraging and motivated me to continue the work of rewriting and completing this project.

I thank Keith Buhler, who provided suggestions for my book structure and opening chapter edits. His feedback helped me to improve my book, and I am very thankful. I regard Keith as exceptional at everything related to reading and writing. His website is www.readingintentionally.com.

I thank my mom for her abundant encouragement and support. Her continued positivity and belief in my ability to write this book inspired me to complete the hard work. She made many suggestions for clarification and editing, and my book is better as a result.

Most of all, I thank God, Who is the reason for this book. God answered my prayers for guidance and energy. He gave me the time and inspiration to complete this project. I believe He brings redemption out of our stories and uses our stories to help others.

PART I: THE CALIFORNIA DESERT

1 A clinic run by a guy on drugs

June 2009 Las Vegas, Nevada

I am 28 years old sitting at a table in a Las Vegas airport in mid-June. My wrist is gliding a six-inch Subway sandwich into my mouth, bite by bite. For the first time in my life, I have no will to live. Not even an ounce.

I'm puzzled by this sandwich moving into my mouth. Am I the one moving it? I don't care about this sandwich.

Now my legs are moving. Left, right, left, right.

Why am I walking? I am stumped. My will to keep going is totally gone. I am analyzing what makes the body move. I think it must be hope, yet it can't be—I do not have any.

I used to love the airport blur of industrial grays and blues and florescent ceiling lights; the sunlight and airplane wings outside narrow window strips; the smell of coffee and perfumes. Myriad people swarming like ants; unique faces to see just once in my life as our journeys crossed.

Those days of loving anything at all are over. Unfortunately, I'm still alive.

I sit down and wait for the boarding call and think about my brother Kelsey back in Green Bay. He was half asleep on his bed this morning when I said goodbye, and he mumbled he loved me and asked if I was sure I could handle this trip. But I don't care whether I can or not.

The cool vinyl seat presses my skin through my shorts. To the right, warm bookstore lights are glowing on the other side of the Starbucks Coffee stand.

The thick smell of dark roasted beans reminds me how much I used to love coffee. I don't dare drink it, though. Then I wouldn't have a prayer to even *imagine* sleep. And the books... I can't read right now, unless it's something related to my condition. Anything that promises my body can change, can become something other than what it is. Whatever it takes, I will do it—sweating out toxins or taking the right minerals or getting a whole new brain. Problem is, I have tried everything under the sun.

Nothing has helped.

My auburn hair is pulled back into a low ponytail. The strands in front aren't long enough to stay in the ponytail holder, so they keep falling forward. I don't smooth them out with a curling iron anymore, so they look limp and shapeless. I sure as heck don't wear makeup—that's unthinkable now.

My black duffel is next to me on the ground. I grip my thighs through my gray drawstring shorts that hang below my knees and gaze down at my navy t-shirt. My duffel bag is full of the same: knee-length shorts, t-shirts and flip-flops. Everything is black, gray or navy. Hanes is the factory to supply all the clothing I care to put on. The possibility of my appearance ever mattering to me again is as sealed shut as a casket under the ground. And yet in my despair, I am able to have a preference: to run into *no one* that I know.

Please don't think about me at all. Please forget you ever knew me.

Only a handful of friends know the gist of why I'm here. My church family and acquaintances know I quit my job to "spend some time with family," but that's it.

I used to tell my close friends everything. But this... this is in another ballpark. They can't say or do anything to help. Their advice would be charitable, sympathetic, and humane. But I'm not human anymore.

To keep myself from their view, I am going to fall off the planet. My parents' house is in Clove Valley, a small desert town in southern California that I've only been to once. My stepdad's job transferred him there just two years ago. It's a long way from my home in Kentucky, so obscurity won't be hard to maintain.

Thank God.

Speaking of God, I don't have a clue where, if anywhere, He is. For all the faith I used to have, I never imagined it would die like this. My worst fears couldn't have conjured up the horror my life has become. Christians say God doesn't give us more than we can handle, but they are dead wrong about that. My condition and despair are far greater in breadth and width than the God I thought I knew. Yet I sometimes pray just *in case* He exists. My words to Him are short and to the point: *Please heal me.*

I quit my job as a psychological counselor at a small private college six weeks ago. I didn't, of course, tell the students I was counseling why I was leaving. They think I'm going for a job in a "different field." What they don't know is that I will collect garbage before ever working in mental health again.

Boy, would it be shocker to students on campus to learn who I really am! If they could see me now—no makeup, limp hair, drawstring shorts, flip flops, and death in my eyes—they'd see I am in worse condition than any client who ever stepped foot in my former office.

For the past month, I have been living with my brother Kelsey at his and Ashley's condo in Wisconsin. At first, I thought staying with them, far away from where this mess began, would help me get better. They told me it would. They took me out to eat and on bike rides through the country. But I slid down farther and farther, until I realized there are only two people in the world I can let see me right now. *Really* see me. And that's my parents.

My stepdad is a successful regional manager for a department store chain. He is the backbone of our family and the only dose of calm in a house with nine animals and my high-strung Mom.

But a dose of calm can't help me now.

Mom stays home and takes care of our pets. They're up to five dogs and four cats. Mom wouldn't dream of having an empty nest. She'd fill her house with exotic birds and monkeys before she'd have nothing to take care of.

When I get home, Mom will drive, cook, and clean for me— that's the stuff she thrives on, no surprise there. What she doesn't realize yet is that I'm banking on her to be my audience while I cry, complain, scream, and shake my fists at the universe. After all, the universe is a torture chamber, and she's the one who brought me into it. Her thoughtlessness in conceiving me was pretty inconsiderate.

Truly she's the one to blame, and, deep down, I know she'll take it. *That* is why I'm going home.

That is why my legs moved me to this gate.

I land in Ontario, California, and get my black duffel bag from baggage claim. Beyond the double set of glass doors, my stepdad is standing outside next to his bright orange Mustang convertible.

He's the only man who would be standing there. I haven't seen my biological dad in seven years, after he and my stepmom got honest with one another that he didn't actually want me, my sister, or my brother in his life. They figured we were old enough to handle the truth.

6

The California heat is thick yellow-white and as visible as fog. The glass doors are behind me now, and I'm in the suffocating atmosphere called "outside." He sees me come out the doors with my duffel bag and says, "Hi Augrit!" "Augrit" was the closest my sister Della came to trying to say "Audrey" when she was a toddler. The nickname stuck.

Boy, this heat's a punishment for existing.

He looks sleek. Mom shaves his head, calling it "rug removal time." She uses a razor out of a hair-shaving kit for horses that sports a shiny stallion on the front of the box. She found this at a garage sale when I was a kid. "They all do the same thing," she justified when I protested she was cutting his hair with a razor made for horses.

He's smiling and holding his arms out to give me a hug, wearing a tie, a dress shirt and slacks. He's on the road visiting department stores six days a week, so he's almost always dressed up. He likes sweater vests, too. Mom's the one who picks out his clothes, but he nevertheless looks nice.

Now we're on the highway, and he's explaining the California desert terrain like we're on a bus tour in a foreign country. On both sides of the highway are hills of rock, which seem to me like piles of dead, dry bones scorched mercilessly by the sun. We come upon hill after hill of them. The shiny orange hood of the Mustang is an ugly color and will be glaring in my view for another hour as we make our way to Clove Valley.

This will be a long ride.

Nausea makes a punch deep in my stomach. My parents and I are used to acres of land in the Midwest and things like clouds and breezes and lush grass. It's hard to imagine those things right now in the midst of this dry desert terrain.

I have no hope, yet I am grasping for the promise of it. There is no evidence anywhere in my body or soul that I'll get better. But if someone outside me promises hope, perhaps I can reach out and grab it. Yet not just any promise—the promise must be from someone who knows people *like me* who got better. There's one group of people who can offer me that hope... if they're still willing to.

Back From Dependency, or BFD.

Back From Dependency is the falsely hopeful name of a drug recovery program I discovered online. BFD instructed me to get off Klonopin, the benzo I was on, by a slow, five-month taper. They said to get a doctor's prescription for a special 20-week supply; each week's capsules have 5% less of the drug than the week before. They talked like it would be seamless if I tapered off slowly and took their recommended supplements. I might have a few "rocky" days and nights during the taper... but then, they assured me, I'd be "fine" by the time I took my last dose.

Well, I take my last dose three days from now, and I am anything—everything—but fine.

Following their protocol was supposed to reduce benzo withdrawal symptoms like "rebound insomnia," the one I have, which can be worse than the insomnia the benzo was treating in the first place.

BFD is about to ostracize me from their internet forum because of my panicked posts that I'm not sleeping—posts that are not good for their expensive supplement sales. Last night while sobbing I wrote them another email saying I cannot sleep at all. So far, their suggestions have been to increase my supplement intake. "Raise the supplements" is tossed around often on the forum by staff and recovered members. They must think the phrase alone has curative effects.

And it makes them money.

Turns out their promises didn't apply to me. I think my brain has meticulously grown metal that blocks neurotransmitters from lodging in the right place. My million-dollar question is whether the Klonopin is really at fault. Maybe the problem is just me. Maybe I have really, *really* serious problems.

And it started nineteen months ago with a troubled client.

One day, after a particularly hard session, she left my office, leaving behind her poetry about wanting to end her life. So wrapped up in our conversation, I'd forgotten to ask her the most important question: *Are you planning to harm yourself before our next session?* She didn't show for her next appointment, and her phone number went right to voicemail.

The anxiety was excruciating.

I finally heard from her at six p.m. that night. She said her phone had been off all day. I asked her whether she planned to harm herself, and she was forced to answer. She said no.

I would be able to document this in her file. *Whew.*

But my anxiety remained sky-high that evening; all I could think was, *What if she'd harmed herself?* Beginning that night, I was unable to fall asleep till almost morning, and the insomnia snowballed over the following weeks. By the time I got to Dr. Hoback's office, I hadn't slept in five straight days.

"I once heard someone say, 'Stay away from benzos,'" I said to him. "Is Klonopin a benzo?"

"It *is* a benzo," answered Dr. Hoback.

"I'm worried about becoming addicted if I take a benzo," I said.

"There's a difference between addiction and dependence," he said. "There are behaviors people engage in when they have an addiction—things like lying and stealing—that they don't necessarily do when they are dependent."

Clearly, he had given this same speech to other patients.

"I don't want to become dependent on it either," I said.

"But you need something that's gonna *knock you out.*"

I really liked the sound of that. If I could just get some sleep, I could be there for my clients. I could keep going in my job and do it well.

He wrote me a prescription for 60 pills. "Take two to four milligrams a night," he said. "That's one to two tablets."

For the next 14 months, he never hesitated to give me more when I asked for it.

Near the end of those 14 months, I learned a few pieces of news through reading. First, benzos aren't recommended to be taken for more than two weeks. Second, a typical starting dose is just half a milligram (Dr. Hoback had prescribed me up to eight times that). Third, benzo withdrawal often lasts six to 12 months, an experience described by some as being "swallowed by hell."

It was already too late for me.

Seven months into my dependence on Klonopin, one pill quit knocking me out. I upped it to one and a half pills—three milligrams per night instead of two—which was less than the four milligrams Dr. Hoback said I could take, yet enough to put a grizzly bear to sleep.

And here I am.

I have just one goal: for a BFD staff member to write back and tell me my case is not unusual, that people like me have gotten better, and that I'm not, after all, stuck permanently in this condition.

If BFD says I'm a freak of nature, I'll believe them. After all, they help people like me *for a living*. If they push me away, there is not a single person left on this earth that can help me.

I'll have no anchor to hope anywhere.

I'll check my email to see if they've responded as soon as we're home.

And that's right now.

November 1987 LaPorte, Indiana

When Mom left my dad, she took us to Indiana, where she grew up. My grandpa gave us a little gray house on his nine-acre property he called "The Back Nine" because it had been a nine-hole golf course in the 20's. The nine acres were surrounded by a wooden fence with a metal gate.

Inside the gate to the left was a park on wood chips. The rusted jungle gym was lopsided and shook when I climbed it. The wooden swings were too close to the ground—my feet dragged when I swung. There was a crooked teeter totter.

To the right was a huge barn on a ground of rocks.

The house sat on a patch of grass at the end of the driveway. Behind the house the land dipped downhill to a lake just large enough for fishing; it opened into streams that weaved around more land and trees.

On a numbing cold November day, Mom met someone strange—not someone I'd expect her to talk to. A guy much younger than her—she was 32—but much older than me. Todd was 19. A friend of Granddaddy's said he knew a young kid who would work cheap, and that's all Granddaddy needed to hear. He hired Todd to mow the lawn, lay a long gravel driveway, build a gazebo, put more fish in the lake, and put another teeter-totter next to the first one. There was always another project.

On that cold day, Todd was struggling to un-hitch a trailer from Granddaddy's Volvo at the gate. He was shivering in a thin, white t-shirt. Mom grabbed a full-length rabbit fur coat from her closet and ran down the driveway. She hadn't met Todd formally but had seen him working around The Back Nine. She was sure he'd be grateful when she draped the fur coat on his freezing body.

Mom was an odd mixture of things. She told people what do to. She made up songs about us and about our pets. Then there were her imaginary conversations pretending she was one of our dogs talking to our other dogs.

She had dark wavy hair past her shoulders, dark eyes, and high cheekbones. For work, she wore dresses or business suits with high heels. When she rummaged for a casual outfit, she ran into trouble with matching. From thrift stores she'd collected men's jeans, fur coats, cowboy boots, flannel pajamas, and Christmas sweaters. I was relieved when she wore anything one-piece because it couldn't clash.

When Todd saw Mom around The Back Nine, he must have concluded she was a pretty woman with odd clothes who liked bossing people around.

"Here! Wear this!" She was getting closer to Todd and positioning the coat for easy draping.

He saw the coat and backed away. "I won't wear that," he said.

"You must be freezing! *Please* put it on!"

He shivered in his thin white shirt. "I am not puttin' that foolish coat on."

"You're gonna *freeze* out here!" She was stern.

Todd *was* freezing. His lips shook as he spoke, and his skin was pale. At six feet and 120 pounds, he wasn't much of a body. His shoulders were like a hanger holding up his shirt. His dark hair was tousled rather than brushed, making it look kind of stringy. His chunky black glasses frames held half-inch-thick lenses. Todd was what Mom would call "cross-eyed."

"I bet there is no one but *you* who would wear that coat," he said.

"Well, okay! Fine! You're being stubborn!" She hated that she was still holding the coat as she walked back to the house in her cowboy boots. She walked faster when she was angry, and her high brown pony tail bounced on the back of her head. Her thrift store flannel jacket was tucked into her jeans' waist band.

By this time in late fall, the sky was often gloomy, and from the gate, Todd would have seen smoke swirling up from the chimney of the gray house.

June 2009 Clove Valley, California

Mom has said they don't have landscape here; they have "sandscape." I remember that, because we are pulling up to the gate, and there is no grass anywhere. Her yard is a big sandbox with ceramic figurines and cacti circled by pebbles. Their one-story stucco house is beige and smooth as play dough. Mostly dry sky stretches over my view. The houses and yards are miniature under its expanse and are baking like clay in its yellow haze.

Things started getting rocky halfway through my Klonopin taper. When I got down to one milligram, hell was unleashed. Every other night, I got four hours of sleep. On the off nights, I got none. In the last two weeks I have only slept once every few days for about three hours.

I have three Klonopin capsules left, each holding a tiny mound of white powder at the bottom, .15 mg—five percent of my starting dose. I have to shake the powder around just to see it.

My stepdad puts the Mustang in park, and we are sitting behind the metal gate. Home picks up and moves every few years when he gets transferred by his company, but some things never change. One is that his and Mom's collection of stray cats and dogs is always growing. Another is that getting from behind the gate to inside the house is a multi-step process. It's going to be minutes till we get inside.

15

Mom doesn't wave to us yet. She's fully engaged in beckoning five leaping dogs to the front door. She won't dare open the gate while they're in the yard. I can read her lips as she addresses them by name, and now they're bounding into the house.

She's back outside and walking toward us so fast her limbs don't stop a moment. Mom doesn't waste time—not even a micro-second. She's wearing her typical men's Wrangler jeans ("They're more comfortable," she has said) and a faded cotton shirt tucked in at her waist. Her brown and gray pony tail is looped on top of her head and bobbing up and down. Loose gray strands at the back of her neck are flying out like she's being electrocuted. She flashes a long and wide smile while waving her arms. She pulls open the metal gate and, as we are driving through, closes it behind us. She beats us up the driveway in her steady speed like a wind-up toy whose string was released. She gets the dogs back outside. They pour out of the front door—they've been pressing against it for dear life—and jump at the moving Mustang like a pack of wild coyotes.

The car windows muffle her voice. "Zoom Zoom! Get down! Down, Zoom Zoom, down, *down!*"

Three of the five are look-a-like strays—large and black with long-hair. Zoom Zoom is the tallest and lankiest. He's their most recent stray, and he looks delirious as he's leaping with unbridled energy. The other two black ones, Fuzzy and Misty, are identical except Fuzzy is gloomier. His eyes droop at their outer edges like Eeyore's, and he's frowning. Then there's Tiny and Peanut. Tiny is large with a gold coat. Peanut, a Chihuahua, is running fast on his short legs, oblivious that he's one fifth the size of the other dogs.

I'm out of the Mustang and standing on the sand. Zoom Zoom, Misty and Peanut are jumping against me with force. My stepdad is carrying in my black duffel, pushing down dogs with his free hand.

"Honey!"

Mom greets me hunched over with her arms stretched out, like I'm a child just off the school bus, but she can't move in close for a hug because Zoom Zoom's paws are on my shoulders, and his spotted tongue is drooling down the side of his black gums.

My body tenses and I hold real still. An extra pang of misery spreads through me. The raging hell within my skin might unleash if I leave it unattended in order to push dogs down. Whatever that might look like, it won't be pretty. I must spare my energy for moving my limbs from point A to point B. The only way I will smack Zoom Zoom is if his saliva threatens to get on my skin.

Oh, please no drool. I hate drool.

He is still standing up and clawing me.

My body stays tight. The words slip through my teeth, "Mom, please get him down."

"Down, down, Zoom Zoom! Down, *down!*"

It worked. Zoom Zoom turns and runs into the house as

17

Mom's holding the door open. She's telling me to hurry and get inside like I'm the last of the dogs, then she comes in close behind me so a cat can't slip out.

"Hi Mom," I finally say.

"Oh, hi, Honey. Man, am I glad to have you home with me." Tears are streaming down her cheeks as she grabs me for the hug we missed outside.

Only half a wall separates the front room from the kitchen, and the family room is just beyond. Other than a long hallway on the left, leading to the bedrooms and bathroom, the main rooms are one seamless area.

But this house means just one thing to me—the site of my continued existence. And that is frightening beyond all capacity to imagine.

"Mom, I need to check my email."

"Sure, Honey! Are you hungry?" She pulls away and heads into the kitchen to prepare something for me to eat.

"It doesn't matter."

"I can make you a nice salad," she says, pulling out a big bowl and opening the fridge.

"Maybe later, not now. Is there a laptop I can use?"

"It's right there on the kitchen table. That's my old one. I use it for recipes now. It works great. Use that one." She points and gestures while continuing her high-speed salad making.

I don't know if my face and voice are sagging on purpose, to communicate something to Mom, or if they'd sag if I was all by myself. Either way, I don't have the energy to experiment with sounding chipper. I sit down at the kitchen table and prop my feet on a chair. I'll be as compact as possible; feet on the floor are an invitation to sniffing dogs and cats.

The kitchen counter juts up to the back of the family room couch; Mom can watch the TV while making meals. The sun is lowering but still ultra-bright through the windows that span the two rooms. Swimming particles of light settle on touches of oranges and yellows. Mom is drawn to Middle Eastern decor such as the Persian rug below the couch and the shawl draped over the rocking chair. The colors are washed out by sunlight, but when it's dark they'll pop out and remind me how warm and rich they are. But the kitchen walls are crayon-yellow and look plastic—must be satin paint—and fat red and green grapes border the top of them. Mom feels that wallpaper grapes can do nothing but improve any kitchen. In fact, the grapes for this kitchen are fatter than the ones in our previous houses.

Mom told me about her new food preparation equipment, and there it is lined up on the counter: a dehydrator, blender, food processor, and two "sprouting" machines—trays of sprouts with lids that spray water.

My stepdad is hunched over on the forest green couch and checking the one thousand work emails he claims to get per day. Next to him, Peanut is curled against Snowball's inflated stomach. Pumpkin is resting on the back of the couch, and

19

Tiny, Misty and Fuzzy are on the living room floor along with the oldest cat Dinky. Zoom Zoom is trotting around the kitchen hoping Mom will drop some salad ingredients.

Cuddles is sprawled like a thick rug on the kitchen table in front of me. He better not move any closer.

"Audrey, you won't believe what I've got goin' on here." Mom is gesturing at the sprouters. "Alfalfa sprouts, mung bean sprouts, sunflower seed spouts... just sprouts galore here. Sprouts are jam *packed* with nutrients. I put them in my smoothies and sprinkle them on my salads. Want that salad now?"

My stomach is hallowed out by a big ball of fear. "No thanks, Mom. Just gotta check my email." I wake up the laptop.

BFD *promised* me, over the phone, by email, and through discussion threads—not to mention in their books and on their website—that I would heal. If they tell me now that I won't, my last tie to hope will be cut. I'll be a balloon floating into outer space.

Good thing I'm not alone. If I'm getting ready to go into space, I don't know what will happen to my mind. Mom will ground me. Hold my hand if I need her to. Tell me it's going to be okay, even though I know it's not.

She already put organic spinach, raisins, and almonds on the counter. Now her arms are jutting out as she tries to open a jar of green olives. Her face is straining so hard she looks like an infant about to cry. Her hair strands look silver against the orange hue of her tanned neck.

All my weight is anchored like a heavy rock to this kitchen chair. My wrists are limp on the keyboard. The only part of my body exerting energy is my fingertips as I type "Gmail.com."

"Mom, I'm scared."

"What's wrong, Sweetie?" She stops what she's doing and walks over, pulls out a chair and sits down.

"I emailed Back From Dependency last night. I think they're ready to cut me off."

"You think they would do that?" She reaches over to pat my hand.

I pull it away just in time. "They don't like it when people don't get better. Makes it sound like their supplements don't work."

"Well, *gosh,* that doesn't seem right."

Her feelings are probably hurt, but I really don't want to hold Mom's hand; all I can think about is being abandoned by BFD.

"I'm afraid they think there's something really wrong with me."

She's back up and at the counter again, tossing salad ingredients into a big glass bowl. "Oh, Honey, let's just see what they say. Guess what I made you for dinner? Raw lasagna!"

21

"Thanks, Mom." She doesn't get that her enthusiasm can't rub off on me.

"Let me tell you how I made this lasagna." She turns around to face me, widening her eyes and using big hand motions like I'm hard of hearing. "First, I sliced zucchini. I placed the zucchini in the dehydrator for 16 hours till it was chewy and soft but *very* flavorful. Then, for the nut cheese, I soaked raw macadamia nuts for four hours, drained them, and processed them in the food processor with olive oil, lemon juice and sea salt. Then, I made the sauce with fresh tomatoes and basil, olive oil, raw honey, and fresh Italian herbs. I layered the zucchini, nut cheese, and sauce once, then layered them all over again so there are two of each layer in this dish. Then I dehydrated the lasagna for 24 hours. Look, it's still in the dehydrator staying warm! Will you have some?"

In fact, I will have some. "Yeah, thanks Mom."

"Fantastic!" She pulls out the dehydrator tray, uses a spatula to put some on a plate, and sets it down on the kitchen table to the left of the laptop.

The density of flavor strikes me. And it's rich. Must be the olive oil and those macadamia nuts. I'm scarfing it. It's gone already. I ask for another piece and she's overjoyed to give it to me.

"Mom, this is really good. Too bad it takes three days to make."

My emails have loaded. My heart stops in its tracks behind my chest. I have a response from Susan, a BFD staff member.

My hands are damp and cool as I click to open the message.

November 2007 Kentucky hometown

Dr. Hoback wrote the prescription, and my stomach was tingling. On his steel exam table, I was already scheming how I might get off the stuff later. I asked him whether I'd need to taper the Klonopin gradually.

He said no, that I could discontinue it abruptly.

I asked if there was a different, less habit-forming sleeping pill to help transition off Klonopin when that time came.

He said that yes, Trazodone would be a good transition drug; it acts on different brain receptors and isn't habit-forming.

Perfect. I'd use Klonopin to sleep till I adapted to the job stress. I'd switch to Trazodone to keep from being dependent on Klonopin. I'd taper off Trazodone and sleep naturally again. In fact, in six months, I'd be off work for the students' summer break—eight whole weeks. Stress would be low. It would be the right time to switch to Trazodone.

For the following six months, I slept soundly every night on two milligrams of Klonopin. On a late May night, the big moment came. I was ready to finally unearth the truth about my brain when it wasn't masked by a benzo. Did my brain have the ability to fall asleep on its own again? Or with a different drug? I was about to find out. I swallowed 100 milligrams of Trazodone instead of the usual Klonopin.

I was awake off and on all night. My flesh felt loaded with concrete, giving me the illusion of sinking lower and lower, down through my bedspread.

I took Trazodone for a week. At first it gave me occasional light sleep, but always with the feeling of being weighed down by concrete. Then it stopped affecting me, and I got no sleep at all.

I resumed the Klonopin.

I wasn't ready to give up on the Trazodone. I tried it throughout the summer, hoping it would start working. But by the end of the summer, Trazodone had no effect on me whatsoever. When my Klonopin ran out, I took Trazodone for three nights straight and didn't sleep a wink. There was a buzzing noise and severe pain in my inner ear. I paged Dr. Hoback early in the morning. He called a few Klonopin in to the pharmacy to get me by until my next appointment.

I picked up the Klonopin that day. Sleep in a bottle.

The following week, Dr. Hoback wrote me another 60-pill prescription, and I decided it would be the last.

I needed to get off Klonopin and just as desperately needed to sleep—I was determined to find a drug that would let me do both. Though Trazodone hadn't worked, another drug might, and I was going to find that drug.

Back at work in September, internet drug reviews became an addiction as I searched for that magic, non-benzo drug. I learned of the various classes of sleeping pills other than benzodiazepines and was determined to try at least one drug from each. I went to the urgent treatment center every week to get something new. I tried Lunesta, Ambien, Elavil, Doxepin, Seroquel, Trazodone, Rozerem, and Vistaril.

One night when Doxepin wasn't kicking in, I drank one beer, then another, remembering that alcohol with Klonopin had knocked me out cold in ten minutes. But after two hours, I wasn't even drowsy. I swallowed another Doxepin, but couldn't fall asleep.

I was drowsy, dizzy, buzzing, and extremely exhausted all at once. But I couldn't be knocked out.

Something was very wrong with me.

A few of the drugs gave me side effects: irritability, ravenous hunger, and dry mouth so severe I lost my voice. Others had no side effects. But none of them put me to sleep. I even doubled the doses on the ones I had permission to. Still no sleep.

I'd use Klonopin every few days to give me a break from the insanity of sleeplessness and scary side effects. But I tried to use it sparingly. I needed those last 60 pills to dwindle slowly while I looked for a solution.

But at last I came to the bleak realization that my fantasy of finding another drug was shot. No drug but a benzo could put me to sleep.

I needed to find another *type* of solution. What was wrong with me—was it spiritual? Psychological? Physical? Father Justin anointed me with oil and prayed for healing. I went to counseling and journaled. I tried hypnosis CDs, lavender under my pillow, numerous vitamins and minerals, mineral salts, herbs and herbal tinctures, yoga positions, melatonin, over-the-counter sleep aids, sunlight, exercise, light therapy, and hot baths.

None of them gave me a minute of sleep.

I continued to take the Klonopin between exhausting nights of trying natural remedies.

In October, one year after my first dose of Klonopin, I was up to one and a half pills a night and alarmed at my growing tolerance. I needed to find another solution *fast*.

I tried psychological remedies online, and some were tricky to execute. I followed a 50-page instruction manual for tapping various body parts while repeating a mantra and rolling my eyes backward. It was supposed to rid me of negative energy and prompt my sleep to return.

But it didn't.

I found a website for a man who used magnets to heal. He said pushing his index finger against his other index finger revealed whether there was muscle resistance. He would ask himself yes or no questions. If his finger resisted, the answer to the question was no. If it didn't resist, the answer was yes.

He said it didn't matter if the person he helped was on the other side of the world because we are all connected at a quantum level. He'd ask his body questions and, by elimination of answers, find out what negative emotion was stuck in someone else. Then he'd pull it out of the person by waving a magnet over his head.

I called this guy up when I was on the road one day. I told him I couldn't sleep without a tranquilizer and wanted to learn his fees.

"Why don't we start with some questions, then discuss prices later," he said.

"Okay," I said. Wow, he was going to do a little of this magnet stuff for free.

As I drove, he asked his body if there were emotions in me that wanted to leave. His body said yes. He asked if I was between ages one and five when the emotion got stuck. His body said no. What about between ages six and seven? Yes.

Six? No.

Seven? Yes.

He narrowed down possibilities. His final question was, "Is

the emotion *lost*?"

His body said yes.

"Was there a time you felt lost when you were seven?" he asked.

Yes, there had been, and I told him the story. I had wandered from my parents' tent at a crowded campsite in the dark. Fire flames lit up strange faces around me. I breathed in the scent of burning wood to a chorus of unfamiliar voices. I shouted for Mom until a woman noticed I was lost and helped me find my parents' tent.

"Okay," he declared. "I'm waving the magnet over my head... Alright, it's *gone*."

It would be $80 for a 20-minute phone session if I wanted to sign up. "Let's see if we can get you sleeping again," he said.

Mom agreed to pay for three sessions. I scheduled them over my lunch breaks so I could drive around town on the phone as he asked his body questions and waved magnets over his head. For each emotion, there was an age and an incident when it had gotten stuck. He said they were gone as soon as the magnets pulled them out. Just like that.

Before we said our final goodbye, I asked him how a magnet could pull an emotion out of my body when he was waving it over *his* head.

"It's based on Quantum Physics," he said.

"Oh, okay. I have heard of that. Can you explain in a nutshell how it works?"

"Hmmm... Um... that's pretty difficult. Have you read *The Dancing Wu Li Masters*?"

But I heard *The Dancing* Wooly *Masters,* and I pictured Native Americans dancing around a fire wearing wool.

"No."

"I suggest you read that; it explains it."

"Oh, okay. I will look into that. Is there any way you could simplify it for me real quick?"

"Um... it's really tough to explain. Just read *The Dancing Wu Li Masters.*"

After our sessions, he sent me a document with the emotions he'd pulled out with magnets, so I'd have it for reference.

I still didn't get any sleep unless I took three milligrams of Klonopin. He may have accomplished something—just nothing pertaining to my inability to sleep. I considered reading the book. Then it occurred to me that "Have you read *The Dancing Wu Li Masters*?" isn't an answer I should take seriously to any question.

I'd remember that for the future.

Muscle testing and magnets were the last solution I had found in my internet searching. I had nothing more to try.

I stood many nights in tears pleading for help before my icon of Christ, which rested inside an antique wood crate. But I sensed I was beyond it, that my condition had descended too low even for God. I'd lost my ability to sleep without a large dose of a heavy tranquilizer, and my tolerance was building. I'd soon require a dose that no doctor would give me.

Not even Dr. Hoback.

I was on a park bench staring at my laptop screen on an overcast November day, and I found the term "benzodiazepine withdrawal" while searching online for how to get off Klonopin. What I read convinced me I had hit on something true about me for the first time since the nightmare began.

I learned that benzos enhance the activity of our GABA neurotransmitters. Our natural GABA activity quits performing on its own when it relies on a benzo. When someone discontinues a benzo, it takes a while for the brain to resume its normal functioning. "A while" often means six to twelve months. During that time, the GABA neurotransmitters responsible for sleep, relaxation, and tranquil thoughts are not properly working.

If I got off Klonopin, there might, just *might,* be healing for me on the other side.

Getting off the stuff was the only way to find out.

And I *had* to get off. My tolerance to an already-heavy dose would keep building.

I searched for help in getting off, and that's when I found "Back From Dependency."

June 2009 Clove Valley, California

Sitting at the kitchen table with tinging hands, I stare at monitor. The black letters are moving up and down and getting blurry, and I haven't even read them yet. They're swirling into the rays of late afternoon sun that is slanting through the room.

Susan is the staff member who responded. She got off a large dose of a tranquilizer years ago. She claims the BFD supplements healed her of withdrawal. Between my frantic posts on the forums and my emails to the staff, I sense she likes me less and less.

Here goes.

"Audrey, I have consulted with Stephen, and we are at a loss as to what to tell you. Klonopin is a shorter-acting drug than the other benzos. You shouldn't be struggling this much. We don't know why you're not sleeping."

I'm dizzy. Deep places in my stomach are dropping. The words "you should not be struggling this much" are flying at me like bricks. The email goes on.

"There is a rehab clinic in Oregon called Lombard House run by a friend of Stephen's. They test for mineral deficiencies and provide minerals and sauna therapy. We recommend you call the owner as soon as possible and get an assessment. It's expensive, but we urge you to go get assessed. Other than this, we truly don't know what to tell you."

The email is signed, "Susan."

The raw lasagna in my stomach feels like it might come back up. Good thing the two pieces were small. If they'd been larger, my stomach couldn't hold them down.

I'm officially cut loose from this earth. The last of the hope offered me has been dissolved. I'm weightless, while also being pounded full force by the weight of horror.

Horror that no one can fix.

Mom.

There's Mom. If she wasn't standing nearby in the kitchen, I might really float away.

Somehow, I'm still perfectly able to be pissed off. Susan was happy to send me sailing. I want to reply to her message. I think this is what I want to say:

"Susan,

You worship Stephen. You believe that because his supplements helped you, they should help everyone else, too. You blame anyone who doesn't have the same experience as you. In the darkest moment of my life, you are telling me you don't understand what's wrong with me because I'm not having the same experience with Back From Dependency as you did. And that I should go to a clinic I can't afford for the opportunity to find out whether minerals and a sauna will help me. Do you have any idea what this suggestion does to someone in the lowest pit of hell?"

I stop. I can't respond to her, or I'll be even angrier, and the anger is too heavy for me in my condition. The despair is swelling, and my whimpers are becoming sobs. The only thing in the world I can possibly grip to orient myself is Mom.

"Mom."

She needs to forget about her salad and the raw lasagna and look at me with those wide eyes of concern.

That's what she does.

"What is it?" she says. She wipes her hands on the towel she's got hanging out of her pocket, and she's by my side, bending down so we are at eye level.

"Mom, there's no hope. They don't even know what to do with me. If they don't even have hope for me, then no one can." My words are wading through sobs and heaves. I put my left hand over my face.

"What did they say?"

"They are at a loss as to how to help me. They said I

33

shouldn't be struggling this much. They referred me to a clinic in Oregon. Susan said it's expensive, which means it probably costs thousands of dollars a day. We could never afford that."

"A clinic? Where? What's it called?" She gets up, grabs paper and a pen from a kitchen drawer, and looks at me.

I tell her the name. "It's run by a friend of Stephen's. They test for mineral deficiencies and then you sit in a sauna for, like, hours a day. I can't handle sitting in a sauna. Plus I can't let you guys spend a ton of money," I say.

"Don't worry about that right now. Why don't we give them a call?" She waits for me to answer.

"Okay. I guess we can call them."

"Let's call," she says, back at my table leaning over me with her fingers on the keyboard, Googling the name of the clinic for a phone number.

"They have given up all hope on me. They don't know why I'm not sleeping. Mom, do you think there's something permanently wrong with me?"

But I already know there is; every hopeless cell of my body is declaring that my life is officially over.

"Honey, no, not permanent. Not permanent. Let's just take things one step at a time. We'll give 'em a call. Might as well just have a conversation." She's already dialing.

"Okay, Mom. Thank you. Can I listen in, too?"

"Yes of course. Go grab the cordless phone by my desk in the family room."

I step around Fuzzy, Misty, Tiny and Dinky to get to the cordless phone, passing my stepdad—I know he's listening. Through the window the orange sun is sitting at the bottom of the sky, soon to disappear under it.

The oppressive sun will leave us alone in a while.

I walk back into the kitchen and sit on a stool at the counter that faces Mom. Mom leans over and rests her elbows next to the sprouters, cordless phone in hand. She dials up the number as I wait to pick up the call on my cordless.

We hear the ring on the line. A receptionist answers, and Mom asks to speak with the person who runs the place. We're put on hold.

It's taking a few minutes for someone to get to the phone. The raw lasagna's still floating up within me.

I feel like I'm under water gasping for air—I need relief *at this moment*. I don't have time to find out whether many hours in a sauna can help me—not at my parents' expense, and not at the risk of feeling my insides bake. Could that *really* give me my sleep back? I'm in too much despair to experiment.

A man is finally on the line. Mom asks him what they do.

"... ...We do... ... testing."

Maybe there's a lag on the phone line. Or maybe he's a stutterer.

"I'm sorry, Sir," says Mom, "But there was some sort of gap between my question and your response. Is there something wrong with your phone?"

Loooong pause.

"No, I don't believe so. I can... ... hear you... ... just fine."

"Okay, then. We'd really like to know what kind of testing you do. My daughter was on Klonopin and..."

I interrupt her.

"I am almost off Klonopin. I was on three milligrams a night. I cannot sleep at all. I am wondering if I have benzo withdrawal syndrome or if there is something else wrong with me. I am a member of BFD, and Stephen and another staff member referred me to you."

Looong silence.

"Yes," he says.

Another long gap of nothing.

"... ... I know... ... Stephen."

"Do you have patients there in benzo withdrawal? Does the

36

withdrawal get better with your program?" I say.

"... ... We... ... have... ... all kinds of patients... We... have... patients on drugs... ... and off of drugs."

This guy is apparently one of those *on* drugs.

"Okay," I continue. "What I want to know is, do people in benzo withdrawal get better? Does their sleep come back?"

"... What we need to do... ... is... ... some tests first. Test for .... mineral contents and... ... get a plan going. How soon could you get here?"

How soon can I *get* there? Are you kidding me? This guy's rent must be due.

And he's definitely stoned. I don't even have to look at Mom's face to know she's thinking the same thing.

She interjects. "We would like to know the price and also the duration of the program."

"... ... She will come for... ... 21 days and the cost... is... ... fifteen thousand dollars for 21 days."

No way.

Mom is going to say, "No, thank you."

Instead she says, "Please tell us what else happens in your program other than the testing."

Long, long pause.

"... ... Other... than testing... ... it depends. She will... be put on... supplements... Then she will... ... sit in a sauna. Sauna therapy."

"How long would I be in the sauna each day?" I say.

"... It... amounts to... about... six hours."

He never answered my first question.

"Have you seen some people with insomnia start sleeping again after time in the sauna?"

Pause.

"We can... ... see about getting those... mineral levels raised and evaluate... after... ... three weeks. See about... getting you sleeping again."

What a hoax.

This conversation's gone much worse than I expected. Mom has to be thinking the same thing.

"Okay, well, we'll think about it and call you back," she says.

Pause.

"... Would you... ... be able to come... this Tuesday?" he says.

It's Sunday.

"We'll talk about it then call you back and let you know," Mom says again.

We hang up the phone.

"What the heck is wrong with that guy?" I say. "Mom, he was stoned!"

She is standing back up and nodding with her inner eyebrows pointing down. "I agree. I agree. Something was very, very wrong with him."

I am whimpering again. Not a chance I'm going to this place, my unrested body in 160 degrees in a dark room with strung-out strangers and no sleep at night to recuperate. I'd never forgive myself for costing my parents $15,000.

I am sobbing. "Mom, there is no hope for me!"

"Now, let's not jump to that conclusion yet."

"*Yet!* You are going to give up hope for me, too!"

"No, Honey, I will *never* give up hope for you."

"I'm never gonna sleep again for the rest of my life!"

"Oh, you absolutely will," she says. "You absolutely *will* sleep, Audrey. That's a promise."

"I need relief now," I wail. "I need relief *now!*"

"I know you do, Sweetie." She's coming toward me with her

arms outstretched.

I don't resist.

After a minute, I pull back and say, "Mom, if they don't even think I'm gonna heal, then how can *you* think I'm gonna heal?"

"Honey, God has never, ever let me down, and He won't let me down now," she says.

Her words are a flimsy shot into a dark canyon. Standing with her hands on her hips, she looks frail and ignorant. The delusion of control is showing on her face. She's not larger than life anymore, like she was when I was a child and looked up to her.

The sun has gone down; the wallpaper border grapes have turned darker shades of green and red. The kitchen walls reflect the fluorescent ceiling lights and look even more crayon yellow than they did earlier.

My stepdad is still on his laptop on the couch. I walk over and sit down and put my hands against my face. But my hands cannot keep my despair from growing. My mental and physical state has no explanation—not even BFD can explain it. They can rest in peace that they've covered themselves by referring me. They cut me off from the only source of hope I had: their promises that I would get better if only I did what they told me to.

The last time I slept was in my brother's bed in Wisconsin. I slept for two hours mid-morning. That was days ago, and with each passing day, the memory of sleep gets further behind me. There is now no evidence either within me or outside of me that I will get better, and no one in the world can help me—not doctors, drugs, natural remedies, or BFD supplements.

The faded hues are gone from the house along with the blazing sun. Soon, Mom will turn on all the lamps.

If I have a choice between the sun beating down and the sun taking a hiatus, I opt for the second one. Let's just say me and the night sky have bonded, after the time I've spent sleepless on my back in the dark. After all, it's not the night's fault I'm going through this. Rather, the night is a blanket shielding me from the intruding flashlight of day. I'm almost anticipating bedtime.

"Let's go ahead and put you to bed," says Mom. She leaves her spot in the kitchen and stands in front of the couch to face me.

"*Put* me to bed? I can put myself to bed! I'm not a child. Plus it's way too early. I'll just lie there. I can't lie there for twelve hours. That's too long to be on my back."

"Studies show the deepest sleep happens before midnight," she says. "You go to bed earlier, you sleep better. *Period.*"

"Oh, my gosh, Mom! I don't *sleep*, so it doesn't matter! It's only eight o'clock!"

"Let's put you down with some Sleepy-time tea and Tylenol PM."

Her tone says this isn't optional.

"Put me *down?* Am I a dog going to the vet to *die?* You know I don't sleep! Have you listened to *anything* I've said?"

Too much energy went into those words—energy that was needed to keep my inner hell intact. Now it is pounding against my skull and leaking out. I press my left hand on my forehead like I can push it back in. My face is getting warm, and tears are falling.

These tears are the closest thing I can get to a barricade between me and Mom, and for that reason they almost feel comforting.

Almost.

Mom always says my stepdad has no flaws, but there's one I know of: he holds stuff in. Though he's knee-deep in emails, he's listening. The tension is building in him, too. I know it. He doesn't like it when we yell. More specifically, he doesn't like it when anyone yells at Mom. I've seen his fury unleash before. I'm wondering how long till he loses it.

On the other end of the couch though, he's calm.

Huh. Well, good thing.

"I'm gonna warm up the Sleepy-time tea. That Tylenol PM is gonna *knock. you. out.*"

Fury is shooting like flames through my chest.

Uh uh. She's got to be kidding.

I want to kill her.

"Oh, my gosh. Oh, my gosh. This isn't happening. I can't have this conversation. I don't have the energy."

Mom walks to the sink and fills a mug with tap water. She turns to face my direction as she talks.

"When *I* take Tylenol PM along with Sleepy-time tea, it knocks me out *cold*. I know *nothing* till morning." She shuts the door to the microwave and sets the timer to one minute.

"Antihistamines *wire* me! They don't work for everyone! You gave me Tylenol PM once in college and I was up all night long with my head buzzing. I thought demons were tormenting me!"

"You gotta trust me on this one," she says. She's dropping two blue gel caps into the palm of her hand. "Just tonight, take the Tylenol PM with the Sleepy-time tea. I think you'll be *real* surprised."

"Not even a big dose of Klonopin would knock me out anymore! That's enough to knock out a bear! You think *Tylenol PM's* gonna put me to sleep? I am not taking it! I'm not gonna deal with the head-buzzing!"

She walks over to the couch carrying the mug of water and the gel caps.

"You gotta trust me on this. You just hafta trust me. I can heal you, Audrey. I *can.*"

Old rage is surging through me and gathering with it every memory of her controlling me since I was a kid. Just as my life is ending, I'm back in her grip. After leaving for college it was easy to forget what it was like being under her roof. It's all coming back now.

I'm spilling enough tears to fantasize that they're a thick sheet of water.

"You haven't heard a *word* I've said. Leave me alone! I'm going to my room."

I push myself up from the couch, wailing like a toddler who has been forced to go to bed. I know which room Mom designated for me because I saw my stepdad take my black duffel in there. It's the left bedroom in the hallway. I walk in, flip the light switch, and on goes the lamp on the dresser—a big mosaic parrot. The shade and the parrot underneath it are bits of glass in reds, blues, yellows and greens. An oval bulb sits on the parrot's head and sends soft patches of color to the wall behind it. The Indian print bedspread is smoothed so perfectly it looks like something from a *Better Homes and Gardens* photo shoot. A rocking chair at the right corner is draped in a fringed shawl that matches my bedspread.

The rich colors and ambiance remind me of times I could be

comforted. I can't bring myself to get on the bed yet; the bed is a reminder I can't sleep, so I want to put it off. I sit on the floor and hug my knees up toward me.

Oh, my gosh. Mom's coming.

"Here, Honey. I have the tea and the Tylenol."

Get the hell away from me.

My whimpering, which never totally died, revives. "Please go away. *Please* go away."

"Just let me tuck you in."

"It's too early. I'm not getting in the bed yet."

She sets the tea on the dresser and leaves the doorway.

Good.

I cross my legs Indian style so that they'll stretch. My back is straight against the edge of the bed, and I need to cry some more. That usually entails me putting my hands in my face, but just to break the monotony I will keep my head back and let the tears stream down and wet my chin and shirt. Though I can't stop being conscious, I can at least try to change things up.

Sorrow rolls out with my tears. Could be my imagination, but I think God might feel sorry for me, too. The idea that He cares, however fleeting, feels out of place here in hell.

That Indian print bedspread might be calling me after all, only because I am tired of sitting here and ready for a change of scenery. Time to transition to staring at the ceiling rather than the wall.

I stand and disrupt the flawless finish of the bedspread by peeling it back. I kick off my flip-flops. As for pajama's, I'm keeping on my Hanes t-shirt and drawstring shorts. I pull my covered rubber-band from my hair and drop it on the dresser next to the parrot lamp. I won't turn the lamp off yet because the rich blotches of color on the wall are pretty. I get under the covers.

Oh, no, there's Mom in the doorway again.

She comes in and sits on the bedspread next to my calves. This tightens the blanket on them. Her left palm is thrust forward, holding the synthetic blue Tylenol PM gel caps like we're in the Matrix movie.

She looks so pitiful in her ignorance. I feel a little sorry for her.

"Honey, will you *please* take these?" Her voice is a gentle plea, unlike before.

I'm getting a little soft-hearted. Must be the calming colors in this room combined with the pity I feel for both of us. Plus, what's she going to do, force the Tylenol into my mouth? Even if she does, she can't make me swallow it.

"No. I'm not taking it. I wouldn't take those pills to save my life."

"Will you at least drink the Sleepy-time tea?"

"Sleepy-time tea has chamomile in it. Chamomile acts on the same brain receptors as benzos, but much more weakly."

"Oh."

"I don't need to screw up my brain any more than it already is."

"The tea might relax you," she says. "Just try it."

On second thought, my brain receptors are already fried beyond repair, and a little more damage won't make a dent. "Sure, go ahead and hand me the tea."

She closes her palm on the gelcaps and leans forward to grab the tea from the dresser. "Here you go," she says with a bright smile, as if drinking it will make everything good again.

"Mom, will you open the right side of my duffel bag and get out the bottle of Klonopin? I have only three left, then that stuff's outta my life forever."

"Sure, Sweetie." She finds the bottle in my bag and hands it to me.

I twist off the cap and tip the bottle till a capsule falls out. There's so little powder in this capsule that it would stay pinched between a finger and thumb. It's too little to affect me, but I'm still going to follow protocol and get off this stuff a little bit less at a time.

47

"Soon I'll be off this forever," I say.

"Yes, Honey, that'll be a good thing."

Her palm is still closed on the Tylenol PM gel caps.

I sit up straight and gulp the Klonopin capsule with the lukewarm tea.

She takes the mug when I'm done and stands up to leave. "Tomorrow starts your colon cleansing at the holistic center."

Oh, yeah. She told me about that on the phone before I got here. I am going to fight with her on this. But tonight's not the night.

"Okay, Mom. Night. Love you."

"Love you too, Honey. See you bright and early." She bends down and kisses my forehead.

She's out of the room.

The scenery in here reminds me of the world I used to live in, back when there was comfort. The world I live in now, though, is a very bad dream—the worst kind of dream. And there's no waking up. I reach over, still lying down, to shut off the parrot lamp.

Its reflections disappear from the wall.

If only my thoughts would fade into desperately-needed oblivion... But they won't. In college, I'd stay up all night writing a paper or having a good conversation. Just *24 hours* of no sleep would leave me feeling like a train wreck. But now... *night after night after night* of no sleep... I'm in an unending corridor, the exhaustion as solid as steel.

Tyenol PM...

Nothing I say can make Mom understand there's no help for me. It is my *body* that understands; my body remembers the many drugs, the natural remedies, and waking up throughout the night after swallowing three milligrams of Klonopin when two had once knocked me unconscious.

Now only an anesthetic used for *surgeries* would put me out, and even if I could get one, why would I want it? I would build up tolerance to that, too, and be even more ravaged than I am now. Desperate as I am for sleep, I am *more* desperate to escape from the chemicals that did this to me. To *somehow* turn around and go back.

If there was a doctor that could help me, I would go. If there was a drug that could make me sleep for the rest of my life, I would take it. But there isn't. My body knows that... a deep knowing, a beyond-a-shadow-of-a-doubt kind of knowing, a knowing that can't be given to someone else.

Mom doesn't get it; she can't. But there's nowhere to go from here, no one to turn to but my parents. I don't know what will happen; I only know that it will happen here, with them.

Which is troubling. My own life is ruined, but I don't have the heart to ruin theirs.

2 The inside of a tornado

June 1988 LaPorte, Indiana

By the time summer came, we were used to Todd. Mom had been inviting him inside for meals. He'd play with us afterward, and he played like a kid. When piecing together the parts of my brother Kelsey's action figures, he wasn't thinking of his main job—bagging groceries at the supermarket—or his tasks on The Back Nine. He was thinking about the action figures, just like three-year-old Kelsey was.

For hours in front of our house, he pitched a plastic ball while Kelsey swung his toy bat. He took Kelsey, my sister Della, and me fishing down the hill at the lake. He taught me how to cast the line.

Mom went out some nights and asked Todd to feed us, bathe us, and put us to bed. No way was I letting this strange man with a strange age see me in a bathtub. So I sat next to him on the bathroom floor as he splashed water on Della and

Kelsey. I helped him wash their hair and resolve their fights over rubber toys.

After bath time, we played Monopoly in the living room. It was a small room, but I loved its wood floors, fireplace, antique couch, and big window facing the lake and streams down the hill. The green cloth of the couch was a paisley print, and the wood of its arms curled into carved circles. On the floor was a large Oriental rug on which we spread the Monopoly game. How I loved the crackling of real fire on logs. Between the living room and dining room was a sliding door made of vertical barn-siding planks.

Todd passed the Monopoly properties to us as if dealing cards; we didn't have to earn them. But this didn't keep the game from lasting for hours. At bedtime, Todd slid the game under the couch so that we could resume it the next time he watched us.

September 1988 LaPorte, Indiana

In the fall, I was seven years old, and Mom struck a deal with Todd as they stood in the dining room. The bright sky outside the sliding glass doors illumined the rooms inside. The grass at the edge of the hill clutched red, yellow and orange leaves.

"Look," Mom said, "You can keep your job at the supermarket. I will give you a roof over your head, food on the table, clothes to wear."

He stood still, and his crossed eyes were obliging like he was a butler ready for his orders.

"K," he said. "And?"

"What I need you to do is get the kids up, feed them breakfast, make their lunches, make sure they're dressed and have what they need, take them to school, pick them up from school, get dinner on the table, and make sure their homework is done."

Todd was wiry, but the bottom of his belly stuck out and looked swollen, like the bellies of starving children on TV commercials. When Mom mentioned she would give him clothes, I wondered if that meant Todd would start wearing something other than his thin t-shirt and jeans that looked like they'd fall off him.

Everything Todd owned fit into one paper sack. He brought his possessions from his grandma Goldy's house, and he placed them downstairs in the basement, where he'd sleep on the queen bed next to our air-hockey table.

Suddenly, the person in the driver's seat of our navy Suburban taking us to and from school was an embarrassingly skinny 19-year-old guy. My friends could see his worn t-shirts, thick stringy hair, and chunky glasses and know my life was not like theirs.

My real dad was the age of my friends' dads. He was thick and hairy and stood six feet four at 200 pounds. But he was not there. My friends would never know him. I myself would see him only in the summers and, once in a while, at

Christmas.

After school, Todd started telling me what do to.

When I didn't obey, his lips tightened and pressed in while his eyebrows arched down and his crossed eyes, despite their concentration, looked a little to the right of mine.

This helped me feel his anger was aiming at someone else.

"I *said,* finish your homework."

"I said I am going to finish it in first hour tomorrow! You can't tell me what to do—you are not my dad!"

"You better stop *now!*"

"You are not allowed to yell at me. I'm gonna tell Mommy if you yell at me!"

His lips stayed tight. "Do your homework, *now,*" he said a little softer, but he was using every bit of his strength not to yell.

"I'm taking it into my room!" I grabbed it and ran. I wouldn't let him see me do my homework. If I did, he might think he was in control of me.

June 2009 Clove Valley, California

"No, Fuzzy, not yours. Not yours. Back, back! Dinky, here you go, little Stinky-dink-a-rinky-dink... Snowball-ball, here's yours. *Here's* yours. Down-down, Zoom Zoom, down-*down!* Pump-a-kin, here you go my little Pump-a-kin."

I know she's about to yell at me to get out of bed. All my life, the sound of her feeding the animals has been our cue we're about to be rudely awakened.

"Audrey, we're leaving in thirty minutes!" she shouts from the kitchen.

My body jolts. Sensitivity to sound is another symptom of benzo withdrawal. But big whoop. I'd be thrilled to deal with ringing in my ears if I could just get some sleep.

In this land of unadulterated misery, it's hard to believe that certain moments stand out as particularly unpleasant. But they do. One of them is the moment of getting out of bed—which is right now.

I'm stuck between two horrible prospects. The first is continuing to lie here... It's 7:30, my back is stiff, and my thoughts have been turning all night like relentless metal spokes. It's been 11 hours; I have *got* to get out of this bed.

But getting out of this bed is the second miserable prospect.

My unrested eyes must adjust to daytime, which is about as welcomed as lights shining into my pupils. My head will spin like it's been hit with a baseball bat.

This is one transition I don't want to spend time in. I sit up and get out of bed quick. I stand up with my hands against my forehead.

Yep, hit with a bat is how this feels. Daylight glares mercilessly into my opening eyes. I'm disoriented and dizzy. I'm pulling the covers back over the mattress and smoothing them out. I put the pillow with its pretty matching pillow case on top.

"Okay, I'm gonna take a shower," I call to her. I stumble down the hall to the bathroom.

This warm shower feels like a thousand zaps of electricity on my skin. The longer I go with zero sleep, the more sensitive I get. But I must be clean; grimy sweat would be an added unpleasantry.

I comb my wet hair into the usual low ponytail and put on a fresh outfit. This time, my shirt is gray and my drawstring shorts are black. A little variation from the navy shirt and gray shorts from yesterday.

"Audrey, good morning, Sweetie! How'd you sleep?" Mom chirps as I come in the kitchen.

I'm already whimpering, and I trust that helps answer her question.

"Good morning," I mumble.

My stepdad lifts his face from the laptop and puts on his cheerful and goofy smile. "Good morning, Sweetie." He has the intelligence not to ask me how I slept, even if Mom doesn't.

Snowball, Cuddles, Dinky, Pumpkin, Zoom Zoom, Tiny, and Misty are in sight. The sunrise has washed away the rich greens of the family room walls and couch. The kitchen table, wallpaper grapes, and yellow paint seem to be miles away. I'm alarmed at the growing gap between me and everything outside me.

"I didn't sleep at all. No sleep, four days straight," I announce through a sob.

Time for my stepdad to leave for work. He's passing me in the kitchen as he heads for the front door, eyebrows raised but keeping quiet.

"Bye, love you," I say.

"Love you too, Sweetie." The front door closes behind him.

Mom is putting kale in the blender. "Well, shucks," she says. "But don't you worry. We're gonna get that colon *aaalll* cleaned out. We're gonna get that *shit* out of your system!"

The Mustang's starting up in the driveway.

"My colon has nothing to *do* with benzo withdrawal! The problem is the GABA receptors in my brain! The

56

neurotransmitters aren't working how they're s'posed to! It will take six months to two years till they start working again! If they *ever do!*"

"Let's see how you're sleeping by the end of this week. Let's just see. Want a green smoothie?"

"Sleeping by the end of the week? You think I'm gonna be *sleeping* by the end of the week? Yeah, right!"

Mom faces me.

"I think you'll be real surprised what happens when these toxins get outta your system."

"Oh, my gosh. Oh, my gosh."

"You'll have four days of colon cleansing and one day in the sauna. Then there's these amazing ionic foot baths! They're so unbelievable, you won't believe it till you see it."

Zoom Zoom is way too close for comfort. He's pressing his wet snout into my torso, and there's already a patch of slobber on my t-shirt.

"Zoom Zoom, get away from me!"

Mom is breaking up a frozen banana and dropping it into the blender. "Your feet carry all *kinds* a' toxins from the environment, from processed foods, from medications, and so forth, and they literally come out in the foot bath."

"Okay," I cry.

"The solution in the foot bath *pulls out* the toxins, and the water changes colors!" She's pronouncing her words so crisply, I can see the sounds formulate in her teeth. She runs the blender then says, "Here, why don't you have a green smoothie?"

"No, thank you."

"Okay, I'm gonna take the dogs out to widdle and then we need to get going. You're appointment is at 8:15."

"Widdle? Oh, my gosh. Please don't use that word!"

"Who's gotta go, gotta go, gotta go-*oooh*... bathroom, one more time, who's gotta go, who's gotta go," Mom sings while shooting toward the door in front of a trail of scurrying dogs. Peanut is trotting in quick little steps, excited about this simple routine, not least of all because it is accompanied by a song he's familiar with.

I let out more tears.

When the dogs are back inside, Mom ushers me through the door.

The sun hasn't been out long enough to bake the neighborhood. I'd like to stand on the cool sand in the front yard before it gets hot. But Mom is getting right into the Yukon and intends me to do the same.

This old maroon Yukon has that musty smell of previous owners and an unfortunate beige interior. It's also caked with cat and dog hair, since this is how the animals travel to the vet. Mom gets out and opens the gate, drives us through it, then gets out and closes it.

Wasted seconds I could be standing with my feet in the sand.

We are on a busy road in Clove Valley. The storefront plazas look like tiny toy buildings nestled into the sandscape, which is blending into the white-yellow sky.

Wow, the holistic clinic is only three minutes away.

A secretary is sitting behind sliding glass windows. I don't know what Mom is going to say, but she's got no filter, especially when introducing me to strangers. On top of that, she has a way of trying to force me to chat with them.

I sure as hell don't want to chat with a stranger. I take a seat clear on the other side of the gray-blue waiting room and turn my face the other way.

Mom approaches her. I can't hear the secretary, but Mom's booming voice is loud and clear. There are no other clients waiting. If there were, this would be much more humiliating.

"Hi, there! I've got my daughter Audrey here for her 8:15 appointment... Yes, thank you... I've gotter' scheduled here *all* week long. Audrey got off a heavy dose of Klonopin and can't sleep. She hasn't slept at all for *four days*."

I cover the right side of my face with my hand because the

secretary is probably trying to get a good look at me.

Great opening line, Mom.

She keeps going. "These colon cleansings are gonna do the trick. Audrey doesn't believe me, but the truth is, we're gonna get 'er *all* fixed up."

Man, does she have a way of talking about me like I'm one of the dogs. *All fixed up?* I peek through my fingers. Sunglasses sitting on her forehead, Mom is looking in my direction, nodding and smiling like she's on the red carpet.

A 50-something, wide-structured lady with brown hair appears in a doorway to my front left, calls my name, and introduces herself as Barbara. I follow her into a very dim exam room.

It's sure chilly in here. She directs me to change into a paper robe in a bathroom to the right.

Man, it's cold in this bathroom as I'm pulling this thin robe over me. A sign by the sink says, "'Life isn't about waiting for the storm to pass... It's about learning to dance in the rain." The quote is on a black and white photo of a little girl drenched while twirling.

This quote is just another reminder that I've fallen too far for humanity to comfort me or God to help me. Dancing in the rain doesn't apply to me. My body may as well be made of steel; good luck getting any positive thought to break through it.

Back in the exam room, Barbara has me get onto a table on my back and position my legs so my knees are up and my feet are flat. Her voice is very gentle. Relaxing New Age music is playing. If I felt human, I'd be calmed by her voice, the dim lighting, and the music. But the cold, cloth-covered table is rough on my skin, and I'm feeling claustrophobic. Nature is my only reminder of beauty, and I need to be in it this time of day, while it's still cool. But there's not even a crack of natural light in this room.

Barbara is explaining how this colonics treatment works while inserting a cool plastic tube up into my colon. She turns the machine on.

She made it sound better than it feels. Water is shooting into my colon, and my colon is shooting it back out with tiny debris of all shapes. The matter is exiting through a large tube at the end of the table, positioned so I can enjoy the scenic view.

I'm stewing about that quote in the bathroom. I want off this table. But Barbara is not Mom, so I must act civil. I'm not sure I can, but I'll try. She's saying that when some patients get their colons cleansed, the walls of their colon stubbornly hold onto unnecessary fecal matter.

But there's only one piece of information worth anything to me, and I'm going to try and get it.

"I was on a large dose of Klonopin for 14 months," I tell her. "I am almost totally off it and cannot sleep at all. Have you known anyone in this situation?"

Barbara is steering the knob on the machine like it's the rudder of a ship. She leans left to increase the pressure of the water shooting in. She leans right to lower it so the water with the debris can flow out. She's got a serene expression, like she's sailing a sea rather than flushing a colon.

"Oh, yes," she says. "I've known several that have been through here."

Oh, *yes?*

"And they got off of benzodiazepines like Klonopin and Valium and Xanax?" I say.

"Yes."

"And were they also unable to sleep, like me?"

"They weren't getting much sleep, that's for sure."

"Really? Did their sleep come back?"

"It came back, but I would give it about six months. It takes a while for that stuff to get out of your system."

"Do you mean that it stays in the system, and things like colon cleansing can help get it out?"

She nods and leans to the right to lower the water pressure.

Now I know she's full of it. Cleaning my colon won't make my brain start doing what it's supposed to.

"You'll be feeling a *lot* better by Christmas. Takes about six months."

She thinks she's some kind of seer.

"You mean I'll be *sleeping* by Christmas?"

"Yeah, you'll be feeling a lot better."

She replaced "sleeping" with "feeling a lot better," which puts a significant damper on this conversation.

"I hope that's true, but it seems hard to believe right now," I say.

Impossible to believe.

It's 9:30 and we're back at home. I endured that plastic tube for 45 minutes. I prefer that tube not be involved in my so-called healing process from this point forward. And I prefer cool air to hot air. It's still early enough to feel some cool.

Mom explains that if I take a right outside the gate, a right at the corner, then an immediate left, there's a park a quarter mile up on the left. She says it's tricky, but how tricky can it be? She tells me to take my phone. I don't need it.

I chug some water and head back out. I need to move as much as possible before the sun blazes its punishment on humanity. Once it's too hot to walk, I'll be at the kitchen table on the internet attempting to find out if there's anyone in the world like me who got better. And if so, I'll learn what was wrong with the person to begin with.

It could be the same thing that's wrong with me.

The sky is smooth as a perfect brush stroke and too bright to be blue. I'm ready to take the immediate left, and most of the houses are one-story. There are no people out, so they must either be at work or inside flipping television channels and wishing they didn't live here. This place is truly a desert, and I'd be depressed if I lived here too, even if I *did* have the benefit of sleeping.

To the left is gravel expanding for 30 yards and ending in a cement wall. Up ahead is the park on a patch of grass.

Grass.

My muscles are tightening from walking. The open air is fresh.

If endorphins are releasing in my blood stream, they're locked behind my sense of alarm. It's too much to grasp that all sleep stopped suddenly four days ago. I have truly lost the ability to sleep.

Lost my ability to sleep? Really?

Yes, really.

This can't be real. Intolerable despair, heavy as cement, grips all my insides.

The cool air is running its soft finger against my face. The despair zooms out, and I have a moment to breathe. I reorient to the ground under my flip-flops. The sky ahead gives me the sensation I'm moving forward. If nothing else, I'll arrive at death one day if things don't get better before then.

The wave of despair slams me again.

That cool air tricked me. Death isn't just ahead—I'm only 28. What's before me is an unending stream of consciousness with no escape. No rest.

The wave zooms out. I see death again, on the horizon like a thick blanket inviting me into its embrace.

I need to move for two reasons. One is my muscles relax afterward—the only sensation of relaxation my body can achieve. The second is that moving through space gives me the illusion I'm moving through time, sometimes swiftly.

Here's the swing set and teeter totter in a bed of gravel and a grassy knoll to its right, spacious enough for my purpose.

I kick my flip-flops off at the foot of a tree.

Now my feet are in the grass and I'm taking giant steps, almost leaping to the horizon ahead.

My Aunt on my dad's side is still alive at 102. Mom's dad is 88 and still going strong. With this heredity, I may have 70 more years of this waking hell. But my feet brushing the grass makes me think I'm sailing rather than trudging toward my 100th birthday. That wave of despair is leaving at the speed my feet are moving, so I must walk as long as I can. This grass is a reprieve from the sand and looks like a patch of land back home in Kentucky.

On my way to my 100th birthday, I may perhaps even heal. But *how?* And *when?*

My mind's spinning like it used to before I found Back From Dependency—I'm back to wondering what the heck is wrong with me. If I wasn't sailing on the breeze with my feet in the grass, I wouldn't have the energy to get back on that mental roller coaster. But the horizon is beckoning me to hope that someday I might, just *might,* discover what is wrong with me. If I know what it is, then I can find out if there's a solution.

My path around this park is getting redundant. But waiting for me at the house are five dogs, four cats, and Mom. And that kitchen chair.

May as well walk as long as possible.

Now I'm sensing it's about 11 because it's getting hot. I must head back before I get cooked. Home now and trudging through this sandscaped yard toward the front door, that despair wave is hitting me again. I come in the kitchen.

"Hi, honey. How was your walk? Want a salad?"

I don't want anything. I feel like a zombie, wired and sensing that metal inside my brain—the metal that I'm sure is there.

"I guess."

"I can make ya a really good one, with some of these nutritious spouts. I can put anything you want in this salad."

"Okay, thanks Mom."

I prop my feet up quick on the kitchen table and open the laptop. Zoom Zoom and Fuzzy are nuzzling their snouts into my side.

"Get away from me!" I push the tops of their heads away.

I'm typing "benzodiazepine withdrawal" into the Google search engine. The only thing on the planet that I care to do is find out if perhaps Back From Dependency is wrong about me.

I can't believe I gave them my money. How many months did I buy their supplements? One, two, three, four, five, six... that's well over a thousand dollars. They don't deserve a penny of it.

Yet I'm scared to death they're right about me.

I see some sites offering benzodiazepine withdrawal support. I saw these months ago but didn't read them once I saw they were free. I figured they were for people who couldn't afford a program like Back From Dependency.

But now I'll see what they have to say. After all, there's a chance I could learn new information—something different than what Susan said about me. I decide to sign up to be a member of one of the forums.

The phone rings.

"Hi, Daddy," says Mom as she's slicing an avocado.

My grandfather's words are muffled, but the inflections indicate he's asking a question. I already know what it is.

"No," says Mom. "Still no sleep. Four nights, no sleep." She literally sounds chipper.

A string of words I have no doubt are obscenities emanate from the phone receiver.

"We're doing some colon cleansing and ionic foot baths this week, and I have her on an all-raw diet."

More sounds that don't indicate approval.

"Well, Daddy, we're gonna try this first and see how she's doing at the end of the week."

Hearing myself talked about is as tolerable as getting stabbed. Doesn't help that Mom talks like I'm home with a cold and sure to mend by Friday. I will leave the room if this conversation continues. I put my left hand over my face and tense up my legs to prepare to get out of the chair.

But Mom and Granddaddy are off the phone now.

I'm filling out the online registration for the forum. For my avatar, I upload a painting of a moon on a starry night, since

I'm committed to obscurity online as well as off. Here's a place to create a signature for my posts; in the signature box, I type, "Was on three mg Klonopin for 14 months. Did five-month taper. On Tuesday I'll take my last dose of .15 mg. Suffering severe insomnia."

Tuesday is tomorrow.

I go to the Introduction thread and type that I thought I'd be better now that I'm almost off the drug, but that I haven't slept for four days. I say I'm afraid there's something inherently wrong with me, that the organization I turned to for help referred me to a $15,000 sauna program run by a guy on drugs.

I hit "post."

Those few sentences on the screen, now visible to the world outside me, give me the sense that I am a human being with a story instead of a freak of nature.

I am nervous about the responses I may get. What will they say?

Now Mom is bringing me my salad.

Eating all raw is supposed to do something like recycle all my insides. As far as I'm concerned, I would gladly trade my body in for a whole new one, and I would want that to include a new brain as well.

What is wrong with me?

It could be a mineral salt gone bad and lodged in my muscles. A core emotion that the magnet couldn't get out. An environmental toxin in my blood. An old medication rotting in my sinews. Hydrogenated oils in my colon. A parasite in my intestine. A vitamin deficiency. A demon no one can cast out.

Was there something wrong with me *before* I got to Dr. Hoback's office, or is my brain fried from all the Klonopin he gave me? It's the burning question—the same question I asked myself when I first learned of benzo withdrawal on the park bench that November day. The possibilities are endless, and nothing makes sense.

The phone rings. Mom sets my salad down in front of me and grabs the cordless phone off the counter.

"Hi, Pam! I'm good, how are you?... I'm all ears... Wow... Wow, you're kidding me."

Mom's sisters Pam and Lisa are the ones who turned her on to raw food.

The dizziness and nausea of hunger would overwhelm me in this condition, so I must eat when the pangs hit. I stick my fork in the salad and make sure to get a green olive, a few raisins, a couple walnuts, and a big chunk of avocado on the prongs.

"Pam, wow. I don't even know what to say... You mean it just picks it all up and carries it out?"

There are several textures and flavors on my tongue. I chomp down thoroughly. If I'm going to get these raw nutrients, I better not swallow any pieces whole. Mom's pacing back and forth in the kitchen with the cordless.

"Well, my gosh, I'm not only gonna order it for myself, I'm gonna feed it to the dogs, too! Are you gonna give it to your Boxers?"

The green salad dressing she made in the blender is a little too cold and slimy.

She's off the phone with Pam. I look over at her and wait for the announcement I know is coming.

"Oh, Audrey, you won't believe what I'm about to tell you."

Something that's going to change our lives forever, to be sure.

"Pam's been reading about this stuff called Diatomaceous Earth."

"Diato-*what?*"

"Diatomaceous Earth."

"What is it?"

"It's from the earth... it's a *substance* in the earth. You can mix it in with your food or drink it in a smoothie. It literally binds itself to the toxins in your body and carries them out."

"Okay."

"It kills absolutely *all* bugs and parasites in your body."

"So, are you gonna order some?"

"Oh, heck yes. Heck yes. I'm gonna give it to the dogs and cats, too."

I turn back to the table and look at the laptop. There are some responses to my introduction on the benzo site.

Here goes.

One of them is a woman who welcomes me to the forum and tells me how sorry she is that I'm struggling. Her closing sentence is, "No wonder you are struggling... Klonopin is one of the worst of them."

Another woman responded. She says I came to the right place for support and that programs such as BFD are a waste of money. She writes, "I'll be honest with you—you are going to be struggling for some time... three milligrams is a huge dose. It will be at least several months until you feel better."

Huh?

So I *should* be struggling?

Something invisible seems to hit me. Maybe this something is *hope*. I can't seem to feel it any more than I can see it... It can't penetrate the misery intertwining through all my sinews. But it's making some echoes as it raps against me.

They don't want money or anything else from me, so I think I can trust them. And they know withdrawal themselves... or they wouldn't be on this forum. They are saying that, someday, I'm going to come up for air, and that BFD is nothing but a part of this really bad dream.

They have no reason to lie to me.

So I am *not* unusual?

According to these women, I *should* be in really bad shape. I took a massive dose of Klonopoin for well over a year, and this total inability to sleep is a condition I can expect.

That I should be in really bad shape for at least months is not exactly *good* news. And even if it is, my physical and mental condition is too far gone to make room for a positive spirit. Nevertheless, their words delivered far more affirmation than I anticipated.

The sun is getting ready to disappear. Mom and I are in a set of wooden lime green lawn chairs on the sand. They've got cup holders for our herbal tea with raw honey. The sky's releasing cooler air. The breezes are gliding around the sandscape like banners declaring I made it through another day.

In spite of the contradiction to Susan's email, that wave of despair hammered me all afternoon. It just now quit, allowing me to zone out. I can't feel anything at all, even the prison of sleeplessness. I'm astounded at this gift of numbness and have no idea what I'd do without it.

The surety of the setting sun is a distraction more effective even than the coolness of the morning. Mom has a peaceful smile as she watches the dogs play and sips her tea. This is a noticeable contrast to her looking like she's on speed when she's getting stuff done. She really does know how to relax when it's the time she allots for it.

"Look at Peanut. Oh, what a *nut-nut!*" she says. The dogs are running in circles around the yard unleashing pent-up energy, and Peanut's running as fast as he can behind Zoom Zoom, Tiny, Fuzzy and Misty.

"He looks kind of ridiculous being one-fifth the size of the other dogs," I say.

"I know it, I know it," she laughs. "He's *so* cute."

An ambulance siren is getting within earshot; sounds to be just outside the neighborhood. It's growing louder.

The dogs leave their path by the fence and gallop to the center of the yard. They put their heads together and point them upwards like a pack of wolves.

They start howling.

The siren and stream of harmonized howls is louder and louder... It's now as noisy as the inside of a tornado.

I put my hands over my ears. I've been around dogs all my 28 years, and this is the first time I've seen them act like wolves. Is this how they behave in California? Perhaps there's something about the desert that spurs them to passionate howling. Or have they heard real coyotes out here and aspire to be like them?

Mom and I turn our heads sideways to face each other. There's no way she will hear me if I ask her what the heck's going on. With my hands on my ears, I make a face that says this is outlandish. Sound is pouring into my ears and through my bloodstream.

I close my eyes. Shutting off my sight could help mitigate the sensory overload.

Like a trained choir, each dog stops to inhale at a different moment, so there's no break in their stream of howls.

They are starting to trail off now.

Fuzzy's and Misty's howls are slowly dying and sounding more like whimpers. Zoom Zoom, Tiny, and Peanut follow suit. Their pauses are longer and the wailing is softer.

Now each of them is merely sputtering.

I can hear myself again. I'm not sure when the siren left because the howls drowned it out. I shake my head and look at Mom. I wanna know what the heck just happened.

"What in the *world*," I say. "Why did they do that? That was literally the craziest thing I've ever seen in my life."

"They howl when they hear sirens."

"They never howled in the Midwest when they heard sirens."

"Well, that's what they do here."

"Are there, like, wolves and coyotes here they are imitating?"

"Well, yes—there are a ton of coyotes, but no wolves that I know of."

"This makes no sense. No sense. That was unbelievably ridiculous."

It seems real quiet now. The sun's getting lower and taking its oppression with it.

Hard to believe that moments of relief are possible, but here's one right now: my face meeting the cool air. The relief comes from the good sensation on my skin along with the numbness, and it lets my heart open a little. I will take advantage of this openness and ask Mom the same questions I did yesterday. I'll hold onto her answers, even if they're as ridiculous as that howling.

"Mom, do you think I'm gonna get better?"

"Oh, I have no doubt."

"What makes you so sure?"

"I just know."

"But how do you know? How do you know you are right?"

"God has never, ever let me down. He's never failed me once, and He's not gonna fail me now."

"Then why isn't He healing me right now?"

"He's gonna heal you, but maybe He's just not gonna heal you *yet.*"

"But you do believe I will heal someday?"

"No doubt."

She must know her promises are setting me up for the cruelest letdown. But I'm holding onto them in this moment.

There's something unyielding about Mom. She's as sure as the setting sun we're watching. She'll sit with me on these wood lawn chairs every night I need her to and not get tired of my questions.

She is melding with the cool air and darkening sky. Her faith can't get inside me, but like the breeze on my face and the words of the women on the forum, it can touch me from outside.

And that's something.

October 1988 LaPorte, Indiana

"But Todd, how long do we have to stay?" I asked. He was driving us to visit his grandma, Goldy. Goldy Morgan lived down by the river on the poor side of town. Her house didn't have a fresh smell. And... she was what Mom called a "hoarder" because she didn't throw anything away. Mom wouldn't go with us when we visited Goldy. She was angry that this woman let Todd's dad take her money and spend it on alcohol.

Inside the tiny house, boxes and shoe-boxes were stacked in uneven layers against the walls. Stuff was strewn on every piece of furniture. Goldy sat on the couch squeezed between stacks of newspapers, her Bible, and a slew of other books and pamphlets that came for free when she sent money to a televangelist.

"Hello Grandma," said Todd. He walked over, leaned down and gave Goldy a big hug and kiss.

"Hello, dear," Goldy said.

"How's the back feeling today? How's the pain?" Todd asked.

"Oh, still in pain. Still hurts very bad," she said.

"Well, Grandma, I'm sorry to hear that, and I'm always praying for you."

78

Goldy's light blue couch was tattered. Stitched seams had stretched apart, and the top of a metal spring poked up through one of the cushions. Goldy had pried a quarter in there and pushed it down under the fabric to keep it from poking her where she sat.

Ouch. She must have had to exert effort to keep away from that spot.

"Well I sure appreciate your prayers, Todd," Goldy said, and I bet she really meant it. "How is the grocery store?"

"Still bagging groceries," said Todd. "I'm hopin' to become assistant manager soon; the manager says I have a shot."

"Oh, wouldn't that be wonderful!"

Todd only finished the eighth grade. When that school year let out, Todd's dad packed up a pick-up truck and, with Todd, headed west. At the end of every day, they pulled over at truck stops so his dad could go drinking. One night, Todd's dad never came back. Todd was 12 years old and stranded with just a few dollars in his pocket. Also in his pocket was a piece of paper with his brother's phone number on it. At 17, Derrick was five years older than Todd and had left home years earlier.

After three days, Derrick finally got to the truck stop. Todd went to live with him and his wife in St. Louis. He got a roof over his head in exchange for taking care of Derrick's infant girl. Todd got a fast food job for the weekends. There would be no high school for him—just working, babysitting, and surviving until he would return to Indiana.

It was obvious what gave Goldy's house that very old and dirty smell—dolls, figurines, dish collections, and... trash. Empty tissue boxes and toilet paper rolls she'd never thrown away... empty food containers.

Above the zillion stacks of boxes that lined the walls was a rectangular plaque with embroidered dark pink letters on a hunter green cloth glued to cardboard. It said, "God answers prayer." It seemed out of place in this house with trash and a tattered couch with a loose spring, and I felt sad.

We said our goodbyes and headed down her rickety walk toward our car. I didn't like that Goldy was hurting. I was also worried she'd get too close to that metal spring. Goldy slept on the couch because she couldn't get up the steps to her bed anymore. That quarter could move and unleash the spring and hit Goldy square in the back. I tried to put the idea out of my mind as we drove away.

When we got to the prettier streets nearby The Back Nine, I didn't have to see any more run-down houses or cracked and uneven sidewalks.

June 2009 Clove Valley, California

Day two of getting out of this bed, and I didn't get a minute of sleep. I'm down to so little Klonopin that the amount is inconsequential. With what little powder was in that capsule I swallowed last night, I may as well have thrown a handful of dust into the Grand Canyon.

Tonight is my last night, *ever,* ingesting that powder, and if gladness was a possible emotion for me, I'd be feeling it. On the other hand, I have nothing to look forward to except the damage the stuff has already wrought on my body.

It's also day two of colon cleansing, and I'm in worse shape mentally than I was yesterday. The despair is heavier than my body can carry. Every moment, it swallows me, and I wonder how I will be able to lay still on Barbara's table without writhing in agony.

I heard my stepdad walk out the door earlier and say he'd be home at eight. In the kitchen, Mom is preoccupied with feeding time.

"Fuzzy, not yours. *Not* yours. That's Pumpkin's, not yours. Fuzzy, *this* is yours. Stay away from Pumpkin! Misty! Oh, here you go, Misty. Tiny, wait your turn. Almost there. Almost there. Here's Nut-Nut's! Here you go! Tiny, Tiny, over here. Zoom Zoom, here you go! What *good* boys and girls!"

I get out of my bed and walk into the kitchen feeling anything but human.

"Mom, no sleep. I can't get my colon cleansed today. I can't do this." But I know we're going.

"Fuzzy, no!" Mom pushes him away from Dinky's dish.

"I hate feeding time!" I say.

"No sleep, Honey?"

"No!"

Mom turns her back to the animals to wash some dishes in the sink. Snowball finishes his food and moves to Dinky's half eaten dish. Dinky stands motionless while Snowball scarfs the rest down.

"Mom! Snowball is eating the rest of Dinky's food!"

Mom turns back around. "You're kidding me!" She bends down and scoops Snowball off the ground.

"No, I just watched it! Mom, no wonder Snowball is obese! You hafta *watch* them!"

"Well, *crap!*"

I need to be outside on the grass, walking. But here we are, back at the holistic clinic. Cold room. Plastic tube. Barbara.

She's nice enough, but I can't cry or throw a tantrum in front of her. With another sleepless 24 hours in tow, this is every bit as unbearable as I imagined it would be.

I'm back at the house after my walk. The oppressive California afternoon begins; glares from the sun overexpose the living room through the windows, and the heat threatens to seep through our walls. Behind the kitchen, the sliding glass door is open to the screened-in patio with a multi-level cat house and some cat and dog beds.

It would be a nice place to lie down for those who can take naps. And that's what Peanut is doing. He's sacked out on a cat bed, his tight-skinned black tummy rising and falling every few seconds, reminding me of thousands of afternoon naps I used to take.

I want to be that little dog and have no care in the world. He loves his simple life in this desert neighborhood. Better yet, I want to be *me,* when I was normal.

Each moment on this kitchen chair, I want to escape from my skin. All I can do is post on this forum. Yesterday, those women gave me the promise of hope I was grasping for. That promise can't make me feel better, but I have the fantasy that it someday will, so I click on the Withdrawal Symptoms discussion forum and start a new thread. I type that I've gone five days straight with no sleep, believe I might be in benzo withdrawal, and am scared to death I will never sleep again. I click "post," and my words appear in blue to the right of my starry night avatar.

It's only been a few minutes since I posted, and I keep refreshing the page in anticipation of any responses I can get. Already in my inbox is a message from a woman whose avatar is a photo of Saturn. She tells me her story of recovery and concludes with, "You will heal from this. I promise. Don't let anyone tell you otherwise. Don't let anyone tell you there's something's wrong with you or convince you that you need drugs."

Don't let anyone tell you otherwise.

Could be wishful thinking to imagine her words apply to me.

But they are leaving a trail of light as they shoot through the dark recesses within me.

Here's a private message from a man in San Francisco. His avatar is his real face. He's in his fifties with shoulder length dirty blonde hair and a Hawaiian print shirt. He writes, "I also got no sleep for days and months on end. Your sleep will come back. It's normal in benzo withdrawal to go for days and days with none. You can go like that a long time, and it can still come back."

So he went through this too. He answered a question I've been silently asking: *Can someone who goes without sleep this long still have it come back someday?*

I copy and paste their messages onto a document and click "print." I get the paper from the printer at the far end of the living room and take it to my bedroom. I set it on the dresser next to the glass parrot lamp where the animals can't get to it.

There the piece of paper will sit as I lay in the dark each night. Their words are trustworthy; they come from their experiences. I just don't know what part of me will have the strength to do the trusting.

Mom says we are going to go to some thrift stores. She likes bargains.

Getting out of the house will help pass this day away; I admit that much.

The early afternoon blazing heat makes the Yukon as unpleasant as that plastic colonics tube. My imagination can't grasp which one's worse.

Comparison is for the living.

The parking lot is as pleasant as the inside of a fiery pit. It must be 100 degrees out here, or it feels like it.

But we're now across it and into the thrift store which, despite its deep musty smell, at least has air conditioning. It's old; there's fake wood paneling on the walls, and the carpet holds the smell of stuff that belonged to people long gone. The sweat between my body and Hanes clothing is starting to dry out a bit. My feet are again cool on my flip-flops, and here I don't have to look down to make sure I'm not stepping on a cat.

I don't like the smell of old stuff, and this is no exception. But I like what old possessions say: that time goes fast, that our stories quickly fade. Time going fast is the only thing I've got going for me, the only sure thing I can count on. If death weren't looming somewhere ahead, I'd be *utterly* doomed.

Here are the creased and worn books. Nothing I'd care to read; fiction least of all. Now I'm at the trinkets, all of which are useless except for these beeswax candles. They're shaped like wooden honey dippers—oval with a spiral outside. In the middle are wicks that have been burned just a little.

Flames never cease to smell good and bring some sense of

peace. My church back home burns beeswax candles in sand boxes and on gold candle stands. I've never seen them at thrift stores before; I've only ever seen paraffin candles.

It's a sign. God is giving me these candles... I think.

No, it's just a coincidence.

No, it can't be.

I have no way of knowing. I may as well believe these candles were put here for me. It's just as likely as if they were not.

There are five of them. I lift one up to my nose and inhale honey and wax—the smell of praying in church. I'm going to light one tonight and try to say some evening prayers. Or, actually, I'll have Mom say them. I don't think I can.

I get a mini shopping basket and place the candles in one by one; I can't take a chance of letting someone else take them. Mom motions at me it's time to check out, and I bring the candles to the checkout counter so she can buy them for me.

We're back at the house. The afternoon has made some progress, but not enough. I'm on the kitchen chair with my feet propped up. Mom is pulling something out of the dehydrator—it's sliced mushrooms, cauliflower processed into bits like rice, and a creamy layer on top. Mom dips her finger in the cream and licks it.

"Mmmmmm... Audrey, you won't believe this cream sauce. Wanna know what's in it? Cashews, organic soy sauce, miso, and olive oil. Oh, *man,* is this good." She is serving it up on a plate, which she hands me along with a fork. Fuzzy and Zoom Zoom want some. I use my left and right elbows to keep them at bay, then lift a bite of the lukewarm food into my mouth.

Man, this stuff is rich.

The phone rings.

"Hi Daddy," says Mom.

This stuff is chewy, too. Granddaddy's mumble ends in a question mark, and it's no mystery what he's asking.

"No, no sleep. Five days, no sleep."

His precise words are undetectable, but their emphases reveal that he's offering a fresh round of obscenities then some accusations.

"Well, Daddy, we're not gonna do that just yet. She's still got two more colon cleansing appointments and the ionic foot bath on Friday. We're just gonna wait an' see."

It's less bright in here. Must be late afternoon shadows. It can't be a cloud—I haven't seen one of those since I got to California. I'm reading more posts on the benzo withdrawal forum. Some members have recovered and are here to help people like me. Some just joined today and are in horrible shape. Some have been members for months or even years

87

and still aren't off their benzos, and among them are people who can't work and hardly leave the house. Most have anxiety, depression, and insomnia; many have twitching and shaking, rashes, panic attacks, stomach pains, indigestion, blurred vision, itching, and ringing in the ears. One poor woman has been trying to get off her benzo for two years. Every time she lowers her dose she has vision problems and auditory hallucinations.

I'm one of the few who has *just* insomnia... I have sensitivity to sound and touch, and my muscles are tense and only loosen up after I walk... but those things are nothing. Everything in my body is essentially working fine except I can't sleep.

Reading about the members' many symptoms, I'm wondering why I'm not more like most of them. My mind is spinning again with the usual question: what if I'm not in benzo withdrawal... what if I'm just a *freak?* I'm going to ask them. I can say anything here; no one is trying to take my money or quiet me down. I start another post in the Withdrawal Symptoms thread.

I have to wait for responses. I eat the last few bites of this chewy and rich stuff. I taste the miso, olive oil and pureed nuts. Every moment is unbearable; that wave of despair is zooming in and out in quick intervals, reminding me of my desperation for the sleep that won't be coming.

Mom is loading dishes just a few feet away from my chair.

"Mom, help. Help."

I squeeze my lids against my eyes, and enough tears accumulate to fall down my cheeks.

"Yes, Audrey," she says.

"I can't take it anymore. I'm not gonna make it. I've reached my limit. Really reached it this time."

"Oh, but you'll make it."

"No, I won't. It's not benzo withdrawal. It's *me*. There's something really, really wrong with me."

"We'll let's not come to that conclusion just yet."

"Yet! Why do keep saying *yet?* You don't think I'm going to heal, do you?!"

"Yes, yes I do. I absolutely do."

She's not even looking up from the dishes to make eye contact with me. "I'm afraid you don't. I think you're saying that but you don't really believe it."

"I *do* believe it."

"I'm scared, Mom. Scared I won't make it."

"What do you mean, Honey?"

"I'm afraid I will take my life if this continues."

"But you won't."

"How do you know?"

"Cuz I know you're gonna make it through this. Ya *hafto.*"

"I don't have to do *anything* I don't want to do!"

"Yeah, ya do."

"No I *don't!*"

I hope my whimpering is her cue to stop telling me what to do.

I'm going to go use the bathroom. It's a good time to get out of this seat and away from Mom. I'm disoriented moving down this dim hallway, and on the left are the washer and dryer behind open white shutter doors. A container of bleach sits on the washer and adds to my disorientation because it is poison and could kill me. The wave of despair is back... hitting me every second like a hammer, and how do I know something in me won't snap and cause me to open the container of bleach and drink it? I feel desperate to die, and what if I lose control over my impulses and do something horrifying, something I don't even want to do? What if I become so desperate that I lose all capacity to choose?

This can't be real.

The promises given me by the forum members aren't going to cut it. Their words may feel true deep down for a far off day, but I need to survive *here and now.* And I literally don't know how I can.

I'm on the toilet, and the cool plastic seat on my thighs is grounding. My alarm at the bleach in the hallway is causing an adrenaline rush, making me fantasize I'm in the midst of an emergency with a resolution coming. I envision myself on a hospital bed with a terminal condition, writing letters to people that meant something to me. Family. Estranged family. Close friends. I tell them they made my life meaningful, made it worth living. That I don't want them to feel bad that I'm dying, because I've enjoyed the opportunity to live.

The fantasy zooms out and disappears. It was nice while it lasted, but the truth is that I won't die from this insomnia, though I desperately wish I could.

I'm back on the kitchen chair, and Mom is pushing zucchini through a spiralizer. The spiralized pieces are falling into a big glass bowl. Cuddles, a tiger-striped cat with a curly tail, is sleeping on his stomach in front of me, head lying on top of his two front paws.

I check the forum and have a couple responses. Apparently it doesn't take long to get attention here. There are lots of others suffering like me, parked in front of their laptops with nowhere to go and nothing they can do—a community built of avatars, words on a screen, and shared commiseration.

My first reply is from a man whose avatar shows him lean and clean-cut with short dark hair. He says, "You are definitely in withdrawal. Not everyone has multiple symptoms. Some just have one."

A woman with an avatar of a lion says, "There's nothing wrong with you. Whatever issues you had before taking the benzo will have resolved by this point. What you are dealing with now is just the withdrawal, and your sleep will come back in time."

I will give anything for their words to be true. Thing is, there is no way to know if they are. Only time will tell, and I don't know how much time I have.

The sun is starting to fall.

It's looking like I may make it through this day. The air will cool down, and Mom and I will get on those lime green lawn chairs. If I can get through this second-by-second agitation, then I'll be touched by that cool air again. Just the thought of it softens my heart like it did at this time yesterday. Perhaps there will be no howling tonight.

Good thing Mom is so close by. What I'd do without her, I don't know. Now she's putting seeds in one of the sprout machines.

"Mom, thank you for being here for me," I say.

She looks up at me and curls her bottom lip under. "Oh, Sweetie, I'm *so* glad to be here for you."

I squeeze my eyes and open them to let out new tears, generating as much self-pity as I can. Grief is the only thing that can possibly wash over thoughts about hurting myself and, therefore, hurting Mom.

"Thanks, Mom. I don't know what I'd do if you weren't here."

"There's nowhere in the world I'd want you to be except here with me."

That's because she thinks she can make me better.

"Are we gonna sit outside soon?" I say.

"Yes, we sure will. We sure will. And I'll make us more tea with honey. Would you like that?"

"Yeah."

Sunset is over now, my stepdad's home, and Mom and I are back inside. There's nothing to do, and every second's dragging. The bleach is lurking on top of the washing machine like it might personify. I can't be alone tonight. Forget the Indian-print bedspread and glass mosaic parrot in my bedroom. I'm going to lie next to Mom and hold onto her arm.

Tonight's the night—the last night ever I'll swallow that pinch of powder. Then the stuff is *history,* and I'm launching into new territory. A territory of ever worsening torture, for sure, but one where any sleep I get in the future will be my own.

All my own.

"Oh, man, I can't stay up another minute. That Sleepy-time tea just *wiped me out,"* says Mom.

Must be nice.

"Mom, can I sleep in your bed tonight?"

"Yeah. I'm going right now. I'm about to fall *over."*

Mom likes to sleep in a king size bed in the front living area so the animals can pile in with her. My stepdad has a king size bed in their bedroom, and whatever animals don't sleep with Mom climb in with him. They always talk about how they'll share a bed again one day after a couple of the pets pass away. But they keep ending up with more animals, not less.

I get off the couch, say goodnight to my stepdad, and tell him I love him. I follow Mom to the bed.

"Love you, too, Sweetie," he calls.

Mom is drawing the ivory lace curtains closed. They won't block light out, but that's okay. Daylight won't come for well over eight hours, which is about how long I plan to lie in the dark. The chance is slim to none that I'll get any sleep. I dash into my room, not wanting to be alone for long, and grab the Klonopin bottle. I twist off the cap and empty the last capsule into my palm.

I walk back to the kitchen and swallow it with a gulp of

water. I know for sure this is the last time I'll ever ingest a benzo or any other sleeping pill.

The words of the forum members are echoing within, and for this moment I'm able to believe them.

The Klonopin did this to me.

I hate this stuff with every fiber in me and I'll never touch it again after tonight. Not to save my life.

Especially not to save my life.

Mom gets into bed and I lay next to her on my back. She's already snoring, and it hasn't even been a minute. But she's as useful to me as if she were conscious; I can hold her arm so I won't be alone. My muscle is straining a bit as my right hand grasps her lower left arm. I loosen my grip a little.

As long as I can feel her arm, I'll stay alive.

To the left through the translucent curtains, the navy sky is dotted with stars. Next to the window is a wood side table with a digital clock. In neon green, it says 9:39.

The water I gulped with the Klonopin traveled to my bladder. I don't want to let go of Mom, but I get up and head to the bathroom. The hallway is a long and threatening corridor taking me further and further from Mom, and the wave of despair is slamming me every second.

Lost my ability to sleep? To *sleep?*

No, this can't be.

The thought is just as horrifying each time it hits me.

I flush the toilet and can't get back to Mom fast enough. I lay down on my back, and with my right arm I again grip her left forearm. She flinches just a little and mumbles something about Fuzzy needing to eat.

Clock says 9:41.

I'm gripping Mom's forearm tighter. The bottle of bleach might as well be glowing in the dark in its place behind the white shutter doors.

I press my fingers into her forearm anew, thinking I cannot hurt myself as long as I'm attached to it.

Mom is snoring loud now.

It's 1:59 am. I nudge her and ask her to pray for me because I'm scared. She licks her lips and mumbles something I can't make sense of.

"You'll pray for me?"

She mumbles again, and the tone is agreeable.

I think that's a yes.

The green digital numbers are glaring, and lighter green hues are fogging around them. I turn my face away so I can't see them.

I'm curious how much time has passed now that I've been lying here awhile. I strain my head to the left to check the time. It's about 45 minutes from when I last looked. The clock's moving slow yet the night is somehow too short—I'm not looking forward to daylight.

But here it is.

Mom bounds out of bed because sunrise means it's feeding time. She's never had regard for those still in bed who don't want to hear her singing. Now is no exception.

I get up and make the bed as Mom sings.

"It's feeding time, Oh, it's feeding time, yes, it's feeding, feeding, feeding, feeding, feeding time." She's in the kitchen tapping the top of a cat food can with a fork to the rhythm of her song.

I stand in the doorway between the front room and the kitchen. Mom's voice provides a familiar cue for the animals. The dogs gallop and the cats scurry from all corners of the house and look up at her with wide eyes and perched ears and dancing feet. Peanut stands on his two back legs and steps back and forth to keep his balance. His eyes are bulging. Mom opens two cans of cat food and divvies them onto four white saucers. She scoops dry food onto each and mixes it with the wet. Fuzzy's and Misty's snouts are up close to the cat dishes sailing in Mom's hands and she sets them down at each cat's assigned place. Cuddles eats on the kitchen table. Dinky and Snowball eat on the counter by the fridge. Pumpkin eats next to the sprout machines.

"Here you go, Cuddles. Wait, Pumpkin, that's not yours. Pumpkin, *here's* yours. *Here's* yours. Dinky, here you go! No, Fuzzy, No! *Not* yours! Just wait. Yours is coming. No, Fuzzy, No! Back, *back!*"

Now Mom is mixing the dog food. Misty and Tiny get one cup of wet food. Fuzzy, who's on a diet, gets just three fourths a cup. Zoom Zoom gets a cup and a half. Peanut, smaller than our cats, gets half a cup. Mom scoops the same ratio of dry food into each dog bowl. Now she's making a green smoothie: two apples, a banana, a handful of kale. She's pouring smoothie into each dog bowl and mixing it in. All the dogs eat on the floor, perilously close to each other and the cats.

Fuzzy, not happy about his reduced portion, is growling over his bowl even though the others are wholly preoccupied with their own.

Except for Snowball. He's already finished and helping Dinky with hers. Mom's got her back to the animals while she washes out the blender.

"Mom, Snowball's eating Dinky's food again! You hafta *watch* them, remember?"

"What? Snowball, *no!* Oh, gosh *darn* it!" Mom turns to face the animals and bends down with a red face and tightened jaw to grab Dinky's saucer from Snowball.

"Mom, I told you this yesterday! This is a terrible setup! You hafta watch Snowball every day! Dinky has eaten hardly *anything!*"

"Not yours, Snowball, *not yours!* Dinky, let's put you up here on the counter."

"Omigosh, now Fuzzy is trying to eat Peanut's food!"

"Oh, gosh *darnit,* Fuzzy!"

"I'm taking a shower!"

Day three of colon cleansing. The novelty wore off the minute Barbara first came at me with the tube. Now the thought of being in that room is completely intolerable. I might have to hold my breath just to stay on the table.

Just today and tomorrow, and it will all be over.

Here on Barbara's table, my thoughts are spinning over supplements, vitamins, minerals, toxins, heavy metals, and everything that might be wrong with me. Barbara is lowering the water pressure with her usual serenity. She's done this a thousand times, so she might know something useful.

I've got nothing to do but pick her brain.

"Barbara, I was on some supplements from this program Back From Dependency. I quit taking them because they didn't seem to make a difference. What do you think about taking supplements? Think they would help?"

Her inner brows dig down and she's frowning.

"Well, I don't know about their supplements... It's hard to know what quality they are and whether they're in the right proportions. Here, we offer supplements that will help your liver detox from the Klonopin."

"Oh, okay. Well, the BFD supplements are real expensive and I doubt I will take them again. I don't think they can do anything to put me to sleep."

"You know, there are some supplements that will help you during this time and others you should stay away from. After we're done here, we can find out through some muscle testing."

"Muscle testing? I've heard of that before," I say.

"I can ask some questions. Then, through resistance on my fingers, I can get some answers."

Muscle resistance. Like the magnet guy who read *The Dancing Wu Li Masters*.

I'm tempted to decline. But, I'm already drowning in confusion, so a little more won't matter. Plus I don't know how to tell her no.

"Okay, thank you," I say.

Let's see what Barbara's muscles have to say.

I'm changing back into my clothes in this frigid bathroom with that quote about dancing in the rain. When I come back out, Barbara says we can do the muscle testing now. We walk into the waiting room, and Mom raises her eyes from her book with a smile.

"Mom, Barbara is going to do something called muscle testing to help figure out what supplements I need and don't need."

"Oh, fantastic! Well, won't this be helpful."

"Come on over to our doctor's room," says Barbara. "This is where the doctor meets patients when he comes each week."

Mom grabs my hand on our way in. We pass the secretary and her sliding window. This doctor's room is much brighter and less cold than Barbara's room. Its big windows on two sides let in the California light and heat.

Mom is looking at Barbara in expectation.

"Okay," says Barbara. "Let's list off the things you were taking."

I name the supplements one at a time. After each one, she taps one index finger against the other one and says, "No. You don't need it."

She starts naming supplements I haven't been taking, and her fingers move with energy, tap, tap, tapping faster.

"Now, our liquid vitamin..." tap tap tap... "Yes, that will do you good... And the calcium-magnesium supplement that we sell?" she asks, and taps her finger. "Oh, yes... your body needs that, too."

Speaking of muscle resistance, my muscles are tensing now—against Barbara. I can't trust her. Any faith I might have put in her statement that I'll be "feeling better" by Christmas has been demolished.

"So you have those supplements here?" asks Mom.

"Yes, our liquid vitamin is on sale today for $42.99, and that's a deal because it sells regularly for $49.99. And we offer a month's supply of calcium-magnesium. That's on sale today for $39.99. We highly recommend this liquid form. It has added minerals in it."

"Okay!" says Mom, nodding and smiling at me.

"Mom, can we think about it first? I am not sure I want to put any supplements in my body right now."

Barbara flinches just a little.

"Okay, Honey. We can get it tomorrow if you want."

"Yeah, let's do that," I say.

My thank you to Barbara on our way out the door is a little weak, but it's what I can do.

The world makes just a little bit less sense than it did fifteen minutes ago, and it didn't make any before that. I lean my head against the seatbelt of this blazing hot Yukon, and that wave is slamming me with the same thought every moment.

I can't believe this is my life.

I grip the upper right handle of the Yukon to steady myself. Just now I remember that this is the first day of the rest of my life off Klonopin.

3 Gasping for sleep like it's oxygen

November 1988 LaPorte, Indiana

The air of The Back Nine smelled of everything that had become our routine. Mom taking us to J.C. Penny's for new school clothes, where she grabbed Hawaiian-printed shorts from the clearance racks for Todd. Ordering pizza and coke and playing Nintendo on Friday nights. Going on family trips to the supermarket, where Todd worked weekends and day shifts. The way our little gray house smelled when all the wood was dusted.

One of the best parts of The Back Nine was its trees, old enough to be large and looming presences. I sat on the steps of the outdoor patio at the back of our house and relished the chaos of wind and bending leaves.

"Neat, idn't it?" Todd said as he and Mom sipped coffee on our old metal glider. Like me, they were looking down toward the lake and streams and watching the wind collide with the trees.

"It sure is a beautiful piece of property," said Mom.

"God sure made this place beautiful," said Todd.

Todd went to a Wednesday night church service during which he "spoke in tongues," as Mom would say. He would tell Mom about some things in the Bible, but she'd say she didn't want to hear about the Bible.

Todd did whatever Mom told him to. He was happy to have a home much different than the one down by the river where he had lived with Goldy and his dad. I wondered if his pleasing nature also had to do with Mom being so pretty, like when she was dressed up in red lipstick, high heels, and business suits before leaving for work. Around the house she wore Danskins and sweatpants, and she looked pretty then too, just in a different way.

Mom thrived on Todd's continual attention, someone to laugh at her "play-on-words" jokes and baby talk and her songs about us and the dogs.

I hated this.

In the laundry room one Saturday night, I said to Mom, "Todd goes 60 miles an hour when he drives us to school." Todd was far out of earshot, working a shift at the grocery store. Mom yanked the clothing out of the dryer. She tightened her lips into thin lines. "He *does?*"

Mom hated speeding and I did too. Being in a car going too fast made me afraid I would die.

That night, I was halfway up the steps listening when Mom told Todd her "whole life" was in that car when he drove us to school.

"Under no circumstances are you to speed. You *cannot* go 60 miles an hour ever again. Hear me?"

"K," he said, like a soldier under her command.

Della and Kelsey were at the young age of trusting. They hugged and kissed Todd goodnight and played the tickle game with him. At eight years old, I did not want to hug a lanky 20-year-old with a goofy grin and stringy hair who tried to make Mom happy. I didn't want him to love me either.

Mom said I could start taking the school bus.

Whew! Friends wouldn't see me in the same car with Todd again. The school bus came pretty early in the morning, and Todd was in charge of waiting with me at the gate until it came.

Todd and I stood on the gravel. Tall grass that the mower couldn't reach bordered the wooden fence on either side of the gate. Before us was a busy road, and across it was vacant land.

Todd thought of a way to get me on his good side.

"My friends and I used to skip rocks across the street right before the cars came. We tried to miss the cars but sometimes we hit them," he said.

106

"I wanna try!!!"

He skidded a rock low to the ground so it bounced on the pavement before settling on the other side of the road.

I had butterflies. This was more thrill-seeking than I was used to.

I practiced while there were no cars in sight. A willing teacher, he corrected my form and arm motions until I got it right.

It was time to throw them near the cars.

"How about that red one!" I said.

"I'll get this one," said Todd.

I squealed, and he did, too.

His rock made it safely across the road not a second before the red car whizzed by.

My heart pounded at the thought that the driver saw what Todd had done. We laughed.

"I'm gonna get the blue one!" I said.

I succeeded in sailing the rock across the street right before the car passed.

We did several more... and then another red car was coming. My rock hit the bottom of the car and bounced off it. The driver didn't notice.

Todd and I went into an uproar.

When he laughed, his mouth opened wide, his lips curled under, and his eyes got bright. I got the feeling it was a moment that seemed to him like I might, after all, welcome him into our lives.

June 2009 Clove Valley, California

I'm coming in from my morning walk and sinking into the same kitchen chair.

Suddenly, I can't sit on this chair. I must get a change of scenery, even if I can't get away from me.

I walk into the front room and sit on the bed Mom and I shared last night. It's brighter in here than in the kitchen and living room—the windows are larger and face the neighbors' sandscaped yards across the street.

I will try to pray because I'm afraid not to. I will ask Jesus to forgive me for anything I might have done wrong. And I will ask Him to heal me.

I get my icon of Christ that's against the wall in my bedroom. It's a large print on wood of Christ of Sinai, one of the oldest surviving icons. I bring it into the front room and set it against the wall on top of a beige cat house. It's elevated enough that a dog won't slobber on it or knock it over.

I sit on the floor, and my eye level is a foot below the face of Christ. Up close, the tiny particles of the print are visible. They're just matter. But His staring eyes are real enough for me to wonder how far away He is. Can He hear me?

Please heal me.

My words seem to stop midair then fall into the crevices of the shag carpet beneath me.

I'll keep talking to Him, though, just in case He can hear me. I guess I'll start with the morning prayers.

In the Name of the Father, and of the Son, and of the Holy Spirit. Amen.
Glory to thee, our God, glory to thee.
O heavenly King, O Comforter, the Spirit of truth, who art in all places and fillest all things; Treasury of good things and Giver of life: Come and dwell in us and...

I have to stop. The mental exertion is comparable to trying to stretch my mouth around a soft ball.

The phone rings.

Mom is in the kitchen separated from me by half a wall, which gives me some distance from the conversation about to transpire.

"Hi, Daddy."

Oh, boy. This time he might cuss himself into a heart attack.

"No, still no sleep. Six days, no sleep."

His muffled huffing and puffing, protesting, and swearing are audible even from the front room. Whatever he's saying, I wish he wasn't saying it. He thinks there's a solution to my condition and that I'm idly twiddling my thumbs, too stubborn to get it.

"Daddy, we're taking things one step at a time... Next week, we'll make an appointment with a local doctor to see what he suggests."

My blood surges. Mom may just be pacifying him. Nevertheless, she had the audacity to say she was taking me to a doctor.

But I'm afraid she really intends to take me.

Night two of being next to Mom gripping her arm, the wave hitting me every second. I'm gasping for sleep like it's oxygen, but it eludes me. I swallowed nothing at all before getting into bed—no pinch of white powder. No herbal tincture. No supplements.

Nothing. Like having no ground to stand on.

I get out of bed to use the bathroom. Green digits say 10:45. Walking down the dark hallway, I'm detached from Mom's arm and feel like a toddler whose parent is too far away. I pass the bleach on the washer. Here in the bathroom the nightlight illuminates pink razors on the counter next to the sink. Back down this hall, my stepdad's sports room on the left has a glass display case of shotguns. Everywhere I step I'm ambushed.

This can't be my life.

I'm on the bed again gripping Mom's lower wrist. Clock says 10:52.

These minutes are impossible to endure. How can I stay alive? I can't accept this moment... An entire lifetime is inconceivable.

I'm closing my eyes in hopes of getting drowsy. Can my mind drift off? Maybe my brain will take a recess... *any* sort of recess, like an altered state of consciousness or, at the very least, some delusions or hallucinations. Anything that indicates sleeplessness has a limit, a point of saying, *"Enough!"*

I open my eyes to the green digits, and it's 10:57.

PART II: THE FLEA MARKET

4 Red from the cold

The sun is on its way up. The dark navy sky has turned azure.

Seven days, no sleep, and I'm wired.

It's the second day of the rest of my life off Klonopin.

Mom just fed the animals. I get out of bed and follow her outside to the glass patio table with matching chairs. She's on the cordless phone with Aunt Pam. I'm running my finger over the black trim of the table waiting for Mom to hang up.

"Oh, my gosh, Pam, this *Diatomaceous Earth*. I'm reading about it, and, *oh. my. gosh.* I cannot believe what I'm reading... Yes, yes."

She hasn't even tried the stuff.

"Oh, I know. *I know.* I mean, it's *totally* unbelievable. I mean, oh, my *gosh*. Who needs any other supplements? Sounds like this one does it all... Yeah... Yeah... I'm gonna order it online. When it arrives, it's gonna *totally* change our lives."

Does it save souls? Raise the dead?

"I cannot believe we found this. I only wish we'd found this sooner."

Will it give me a new brain?

I'm fidgety and feel like death itself is wrapped around every cell of my body.

"Okay, well I gotta go. I'm gonna finish reading the paper, then I'm gonna get Audrey to her last colon cleanse. Tomorrow's her sauna and ionic foot bath... Yep, we're getting those toxins outta her system day by day... Okay, talk to you later, Pam."

I have her attention.

"Mom, I'm alarmed."

She looks at me, but her eyes have no expression.

"I didn't sleep at all last night," I say.

"No sleep, huh?"

"No sleep. Seven days. Mom, I'm seriously worried about myself."

"Yeah," she says, still no expression.

My stomach drops.

On this side of the yard are looming pine trees pushing shafts of cool air in our direction as the wind blows through their branches. The newspaper in her hand, iced tea, and glass table are like objects from a previous life. Every molecule of this yellow air is filled with my alarm at being trapped in this skin. I elevate my legs onto the table.

Whatever is wrong with my body seems to be growing like an environmental threat. Untamable. Unfixable. It should be removed from society. And I'm the one in it, its helpless victim.

But no one will put a stop to it. And it won't put a stop to itself—it's not dying.

What am I going to do?

On The Back Nine, I dreamed of being a dancer, a rock star, a writer, and then a professional basketball player. I thought there was a plan, a purpose for my life. It turns out God's plan for me was unending torment beyond anything my imagination could have conjured. I'm being punished. After all, I have been a jerk to Della, Kelsey, and Mom; I was mean to Todd. And this is God's way of telling me my existence has been an offense.

Todd... I hope I didn't wound him for life.

God's plan is for me to die. But He doesn't have the

compassion to kill me. He'll drive me to the point of doing it myself because that's *part* of the plan. He wants to torment my friends and family.

I get it now.

Mom and I are at the clinic waiting for the final appearance of Barbara in the doorway. As my breath travels into my nostrils and my stomach rises, my fate stands frozen in view. It's ironic, where I am, because the state of my colon is utterly irrelevant. My soul and body have already been sentenced, but we're pretending there is something that can be done to help me. Poor Mom doesn't know the final verdict yet; she still thinks she can heal me; she still thinks God has a good plan.

She'll know the truth soon enough though. My body isn't fit for any semblance of a normal life. I'll drive Mom to her grave and eat away her and my stepdad's resources in the process. It's not a life *worth* living for me or them, and the unceasing torment makes it impossible for me to live it.

No one thought God's plan would be this. But it is, and I'm a casualty. My life is meant to teach others something. Once I die, those who knew me will finally learn that life is sometimes too much to bear, that no one can expect everyone to bear it. People will learn compassion. They'll learn that God doesn't always intend to come through. Their worlds will turn upside down.

Tears are sliding down my cheeks. I can still *feel;* at least that can't be taken from me. I put my right hand on the side of my face, my elbow resting on the armchair. This shields me best as possible from the secretary; I can't let her hear what I'm about to say.

"Mom."

She puts down her book and sees my tears, my hand on my face, and my sad expression. She puts her right hand on my left and looks at me like she'll give up anything, everything, for me.

"Yes, Honey."

"I think it's God's plan for me to take my life."

She shakes her head back and forth slowly as if to say no, it's not His plan.

"Do you think that's His plan?" I say.

"No." She squeezes her eyes, and tears fall down and hit her lips.

"I think it's been His plan all along."

Her lips turn down and tremble. She's still shaking her head, but not like she's trying to persuade me.

"Yes, I think it is," I nod. "I think that's what He wants. He intends to teach people something."

118

Barbara appears in the doorway.

"Mom, I don't think I can go in there," I whisper.

"Just one more day," she whispers back.

Barbara saunters over to us. Mom looks up at her and says, "Rough day here."

Barbara can see that.

I follow her into the colonics room, though, because I might as well go through the motions—there's no reason not to. Barbara is snapping on her rubber gloves. She would probably rather stab me than insert a tube into my colon, but that could just be my imagination.

What I know for sure is this is the fourth and last colon cleanse of my life. Tomorrow I will sit in a sauna and put my feet in a bath.

The phone rings. It's Aunt Lisa.

"Hi, Lisa... Oh, yes, I am gonna order some of that Diatomaceous Earth... Yes. Yes... Uh huh..."

We just returned from the clinic. I took my usual walk because feeling my feet on the grass is what I need to do while I still exist. I must move, move, move. Now I'm back at the kitchen table and addicted to this benzodiazepine withdrawal forum. It's my only contact with peers and the only place where no one thinks I'm an outcast or even abnormal. I have a group of regular visitors to my posts, and in return I read and respond to theirs, though all I have to say right now is that I'm sorry for what they are going through. I don't have any hope to offer.

I just found a thread titled "Recovery Stories."

"U-huh... u-huh... Listen, Lisa, you won't believe what I just read. I found out cashews may not be *raw*... The whole food stores *say* they're raw, but there is really *no* guarantee unless you write to the manufacturer. So guess what I did? I wrote to the manufacturer! And he wrote back! He said he cannot guarantee the processing temperature is below 110... Can you *believe* that? I'm not gonna buy *any* more cashews. I mean, *no way!*"

The midday sun's rays shoot through the kitchen where Mom is pacing back and forth with her hair in its usual loop on top of her head, gray stands flying down her neck. Her facial expression says she's on a mission to murder the manufacturers of heated cashews. Her Goodwill khaki shorts end above her knees, and from there, blue-green veins trail down her pale calves.

The first recovery story on the forum is a woman who was on Ambien and tapered off. So far, her story sounds like mine except that Ambien is weaker than any benzo from what I've read. Like me, she went days at a time with no sleep. All of her natural sleep came back nine months after she quit taking the Ambien.

"Really... Oat groats?... If they cannot *guarantee* me they were processed at less than 110 degrees, I'm not gonna buy 'em, simple as that... Yes, that's *right!* I'm gonna see if it *sprouts! That's* what I'm gonna do! If it doesn't sprout, it's not raw. *Period."*

Mom finally gets off the phone.

"Audrey, Lisa says these oat groats may not be raw. But I'm gonna find out. I'm gonna put some groats in my sprout machine. If they *don't* sprout, they're *not* raw."

"Good idea, Mom."

This woman on the forum had insomnia much like mine, and she recovered. But her brain probably had a better shot than mine does—she wasn't on a dose heavy enough to knock out a large mammal.

Mom is dropping oat groats into three square trays in her sprouter. She closes the lid. The machine is connected to a black hose and a timer. Mom attaches the hose to the kitchen sink and turns on the faucet. The holes in the plastic lid spray water onto the seeds every half hour.

An endless string of tormenting minutes stretches ahead, and I have no desire to get through the one I'm in right now. I'm starting a new discussion thread. I type that I've gone seven days with no sleep and that my brain is probably fried beyond recovery because of how much Klonopin I was on. I hit "post."

I'm sitting and waiting for responses. I refresh the page over and over.

Here's one.

"Seven days—no sleep? Wow, after I quit Lunesta I went two days with none then crashed on the third night."

Lucky you.

Here's a reply from a man who was on a cocktail of drugs for many years before tapering off, one of them a relatively large dose of Ativan.

"I got half an hour sleep per night for three years. It was utter hell. Now I sleep better than I did before I went through that nightmare."

Whoa.

He goes on to say he used to sit on his porch and cry out for help to anyone within earshot. He says he is having trouble not resenting the many years of life the drugs stole from him when he was on them, not to mention the three years in withdrawal when he discontinued them.

If *he* healed, there might even be hope for me.

Since I can't get through morning prayers, I may as well see where the nearest church is. I can try sitting in a service. If I can endure it till the end, I can take communion.

The Internet shows the nearest Orthodox Church is in a neighboring town.

"Mom, this Sunday, will you drive me to a church in La Joleta? It's about 20 minutes away. You can come with me. Or maybe drop me off?"

The Orthodox Church I joined a few years ago is very different from the churches Mom used to take us to. Nowadays she settles for sermons on the radio. But I think she'll be willing to drive me to church if I ask her to.

"Sure, Honey, sure. What time's the service? From when to when?"

"From 9:30 until about 11 or 11:30. I might stay after and see if I can talk to the priest about praying for me."

"Well, I may have to drop you off. The dogs can't be alone for more than two hours, so I'll hafta come back here and let them out to widdle, then come back and get you."

"Okay."

Eight days, no sleep. Third day off Klonopin. Fifth day eating only raw food. Last and final day at the holistic clinic.

Today, I won't be in a cold, dim room. A cheerful brunette comes over to Mom and me in the waiting room and says her name is Casey and that I must be Audrey. She beckons us to follow her past the secretary and into a room on the right.

Mom, of course, tells Casey that I haven't slept in eight days.

Casey gasps and then instructs me to strip off my clothes except for the bathing suit I was told to wear under my t-shirt and shorts. The "sauna" is not a hot room with wood siding, as I'd envisioned, but a standing rectangular structure the size of a portable potty. It's covered with tarp, and she pulls the front over and asks me to sit inside. Casey cranks up the heat with a knob on the wall and closes the tarp "door" over me. It has a little plastic window so I can see out.

I'm sitting on a seat not unlike a toilet. The heat's getting so intense so quickly, I know right off the bat this is going to be intolerable. My body is already wired from being perpetually awake, and now a zombie-like electrical current is racing through my veins from the heat.

"How long am I going to be in here?" I call out to Casey.

"Well, I plan to have you in there 45 minutes," she answers back through the plastic window. "We can break it up if you'd like."

"Okay, thanks. I might need to do that."

"I'll come check on you in about 20 minutes to see how you are doing." Her voice fades as she retreats. She's out the door.

Mom is staying in the room with me for consolation. She's sitting in one of the leather-seat chairs against the wall, absorbed with her book on wheat grass.

"Mom," I plead, hoping she can hear me. I don't have the energy to shout.

"Sweetie, how are you?" She puts her book down.

"Miserable. It's so hot in here. It's hard to tolerate this heat."

Not to mention the ambiance—a scenic view of tarp on all sides except for this piece of thick and warped plastic through which Mom is visible.

"Oh, *man*. Think you're gonna be okay?" She's loud enough that I am sure everyone in the clinic can hear her.

"I don't know. Fifteen minutes is maybe all I can do. I don't know about 20."

"Do what you can," Mom says. "When you've had enough, let me know, and we'll just stop the sauna."

My warm sweat meets the hot air, and the resulting steam is burning my skin.

After who knows how long, the door opens; it must be Casey checking on me. "How's it going in there? Need a break?"

I can't see her but her voice is close by. "Yeah," I say. "I don't think I can do any more today."

A loud click sounds as she turns off the heat with the wall knob. She pulls back the tarp door, and a rush of cool air sweeps toward me.

"I'll leave the room to let you get changed into your clothes, and then we'll do the foot bath," she says.

125

I'm outside the tarp and back in room temperature, and my body feels like it's been deep fried on the inside. I shiver and pull my dry clothes over my damp bathing suit.

Casey comes in and puts a foot bath on the floor in front of a chair. She turns on a faucet, which feeds water to the bath through a hose. Mom looks up from her book to watch Casey twist off a cap and pour solution into the bath.

This is the only part of the week I've been semi-curious about.

"So, this solution is going to pull toxins out of my body?"

"Yep."

"And the color of the water will tell you what toxins are coming out?"

"There are several colors, and each one can represent many different toxins, so we will take a look after about thirty minutes."

The foot bath is full.

"Okay, here you go," Casey says. "You can sit right down here and put your feet in. I'll be back to check on you in a bit."

"Okay, thank you."

This is the least unpleasant experience here so far. I used to love the feel of warm water on my skin and wish I could appreciate it now. It's been two minutes, and the water is getting slightly yellow… now a little darker yellow. It's slowly turning into a light brown. Now the brown's getting darker… a dark muddy brown.

Guess I have a lot of toxins. *Or* the solution is turning brown from the dirt on my feet.

It's been thirty minutes, and Casey comes back in the room. "How are we doing in here?" she says. She comes over to the bath and glances at the water.

"It was yellow, and now it's so dark it's almost black. Does that mean I got rid of a lot of toxins?"

"Yeah, some toxins certainly came out in that water."

"Is there a way to tell which ones?"

"Well, the yellow you saw at first would mean your kidney and bladder released some. When it turned more of the brown color, your liver was being detoxed."

"Okay. So is there a way to know what toxins were coming out?"

"There's no way to know for sure which toxins are releasing… the colors don't necessarily tell us that."

"Do heavy metals come out too, not just toxins?"

"Yes, heavy metals are indicated by the darker brown and even black I can see in this foot bath. I bet some mercury came out."

My flip flops back on, Mom and I are in front of the secretary now, standing with Casey to say our goodbyes. Barbara is nearby and comes over.

I un-sag my eyes and lips to even out my face. Barbara gives a friendly expression, and I thank her for her help and force a slight smile. Putting on a face appropriate for the land of the living is feeling as easy as moving a boulder. Mom is subdued, unlike on Monday when she bounded in here believing this place was going to heal me. She hands the credit card to the secretary to get it swiped for who knows how much.

Sadness and guilt jab into a deep hollow of my stomach.

"How are you feeling?" the secretary asks me.

"Not too great," I say.

"I am sorry to hear that. Hope that you feel better soon."

"Audrey's still not sleeping, but we're gonna keep her on a raw food diet and expect a turn-a-round here soon," says Mom.

There wasn't a lot of enthusiasm in her voice when she said "turn-a-round" though. We leave the glass doors of the holistic clinic behind and move into the yellow blend of sky and sand then climb into the Yukon. I grip the beige handle.

A slow death is traveling across Mom's pupils, and her face is blank as she stares at the sandscape over her steering wheel.

Things didn't go how Mom thought they would. If her hope is really dying, then I'm the one killing it.

February 1989 LaPorte, Indiana

On a winter day I said to Mom, "Todd taught me to skip rocks across the street when cars are coming."

She had a word with him. After she did, I knew I'd hurt Todd deep down. I had gone behind his back and betrayed him.

Evenings at 8:30, when the sun was down and the living room was lit by fireplace flames, everyone but me kissed and hugged Todd. It was time for us to say, "G'night, love you" to each other, one by one. When it was my turn to say it to Todd, I stood tense and said, "G'night, Todd" without the "love you" part. Sometimes I added, "See you in the morning" because it sounded friendlier.

I'd leap up the narrow stairwell to my bedroom. Both sides of my ceiling slanted down to the floor, giving my room the shape of a triangle. I would get onto my mattress and tuck my face against the ceiling wall and breathe a sigh of relief that the time of saying goodnight was over.

I would not give in.

I started telling Todd, "You are not my Dad!" even in front of Mom. I didn't want to do what Todd said during homework and chores. I didn't think I should have to.

Something snapped inside of Todd. We knew this on a winter night with the ground covered in a thick layer of snow. By the time I knew what was happening, Todd had his things packed in the back of the Suburban. He'd packed them that day when I was at school.

Todd said he was leaving and went out the front door. Mom followed him and protested. Della, Kelsey and I joined them. He told Mom that she would need to take him back to Goldy's. The five of us stood there shivering.

Mom turned to me and said, "You are *ruining* our lives!"

Her words hit me like stones. Her mascara trailed down her cheeks inside her teardrops. Todd was crying, too; the first time I'd ever seen him cry. He cried just as he played—like a child.

"Todd is getting ready to leave us! No, *no,* Todd, don't leave!" she said, turning away from me to face him. Her stomach heaved deeply, and rhythmic wails came from her mouth.

Her accusation wasn't fair. An eight-year-old couldn't ruin the lives of two adults and two children.

But they all believed I could.

Todd really *was* getting ready to leave.

I panicked.

"Todd, please don't leave!" I said.

"You are so *mean* to him!" Mom said. "He can't live like this! *We* can't live like this!"

"He is not my dad! But he can *still stay!* It's just that he's not my dad! That doesn't mean I hate him!"

"No, Todd, don't go!" yelled Della, hugging Todd around his legs. Kelsey was sobbing next to her.

"I can't stay here." Todd shook his head. He paced toward the Suburban.

"Quit *saying* that! Todd, *please* stay!" Mom begged through her wailing and put on her saddest and most helpless face.

Mom faced me again. "Look what you are *doing* to us! To this *family!*"

I started crying, too. "I am *not ruining* your lives! Todd, please don't run away! I am sorry I got you into trouble! I *like* skipping rocks! I won't get you into trouble anymore!"

"Todd is *family!* He is our *family!* You can't *treat* him that way!"

Todd opened the passenger door of the Suburban. The light kicked on inside the vehicle, then Todd's silhouette disappeared in the dark as he climbed in and closed the door. The Suburban window was down just a crack.

"Todd! Todd!" Kelsey's sobs were desperate.

"Todd," I said, "I promise I will stop being mean to you!

131

Please stay! I don't hate you! I *promise* I don't hate you!"

I was not ready to say I loved him.

Somehow, within ten minutes, the Suburban was vacant—Todd wasn't in it. The five of us were wrapped in a large hug, our arms stretched around each other in a circle as we whimpered.

Todd seemed like a large kid who'd decided not to run away after all. Mom was saying The Back Nine was his home. Our wet cheeks were red from the cold.

June 2009 Clove Valley, California

Mom makes me a salad. My shorts are baggier, and when I pass mirrors and turn to the side, I look a little slimmer.

Not that I care. I'm only doing the raw diet thing to, as Mom said, get the "shit" out of my system.

She turns on the television, and Little House on the Prairie is playing. Laura, Mary and Carrie Ingalls seem so carefree. They have manageable problems and challenges—kind of like people who are learning to dance in the rain rather than wait for the storm to pass.

I'd do anything to be one of them. The show will be playing for another 45 minutes.

I don't have an appetite, but if I don't eat this salad my stomach might start gnawing painfully, and I can't bear that on top of this zombie-like wiring in my body. Little House gives me something concrete to get through. Eyes on the black and white screen, I lift a bite of salad up to my mouth. The fork is midway between the bowl and my mouth. On it are lettuce, raisins, two Kalamata olives, and a few walnuts. I have no motivation to move the fork into my mouth.

I do it anyway, chomping the flavors between my teeth.

The phone rings and Mom picks up the cordless.

"Hi, Daddy... No. Eight days, no sleep."

Here we go again.

This present moment is torment beyond expression. A thousand strings of more moments like these are *unimaginable*. Making it through the entire rest of this *day?*

It's overwhelming enough to commit to existing for the rest of this Little House on the Prairie episode.

Stay alive through this episode. Just stay alive.

That's 45 minutes away. The sound of television inside on a summer day always did make me restless for evening. The sun's full blaze through the windows hits me face on.

"Well, Daddy, I had her at a clinic all week to do some detoxing... ... I know, I know... Well, like I said, we're gonna get her to a doctor here soon."

133

Like hell we are.

My cell phone rings from my bedroom dresser, and I get up and jog to my room. In all likelihood, I won't answer. I haven't been on my cell phone since the day I flew here to California, other than to answer when Marcia called. Marcia is from my church, and I felt like I could tell her my condition without being judged.

"Father Justin" is glowing in white letters on the screen. I guess I care to talk to him, but he is the only one.

"Hello?" I say.

"Audrey!"

"Hi, Father Justin. Thanks for calling me."

"Audrey, we haven't forgotten about you here. How are you doing?"

"Not good."

"Things aren't going so well?"

"I haven't slept in eight days."

"Oh, Audrey. Oh, my *goodness*. Lord, have *mercy!* Are you going to go see a doctor?"

"I've been to doctors at least 15 times, probably closer to 20, before I came here. There's nothing they can do."

"This sounds *dangerous,* Audrey. Think you might visit a doctor there in California? You know, just to get a second opinion?"

"I already tried all the drugs for sleep. I'm off Klonopin now, so if the withdrawal goes away, I could get better."

Could. But probably not.

"Okay, well, Audrey, God *bless* you. We're praying for you at church."

"Oh... thank you so much... But, I don't want people to know what is wrong with me. Is my name being mentioned in the liturgy?"

"Yeah, we mention your name every Sunday, along with others who are ill. We want to keep praying for you. You really *need* it!"

This blows my fantasy of living in obscurity.

"Oh, okay, thanks so much. I just feel self-conscious and don't want people at church to know what I'm going through."

"Audrey, we just really *care* about you. I won't give details if you don't want me to. I've gotten emails from some families; they wanted to know if there is anything they can do to help."

"Okay, thank you. There's nothing they can do except pray."

Unfortunately, when they pray for me, they are reminded

that I exist.

Please just forget about me, because I'll never make it back to Kentucky.

"Father Justin, I have a question about prayer if that's okay."

"Yeah, yeah, go ahead."

"I tried to do morning prayers but don't feel like I can. It takes too much mental energy to say the prayers, and I feel like God can't hear me, and I am afraid I will start to hate praying and not want anything to do with it."

"Oh, of course, of course. Audrey, give yourself a *break*. In your condition, all you can do is say, "Lord have mercy." Sometimes all we can do is cry out. In your state, your mind isn't going to be able to function. Just say "Lord have mercy" at this point."

"Okay, thanks so much. That helps. You are right; I think that's all I can do... Hold on... Mom can you turn down the vacuum? *I can't hear!*"

"Audrey, I'm just on my way out the door... I wanted to say we love you and haven't forgotten about you. Stay in touch, okay?"

"Okay, thank you so much for calling."

"Don't be a stranger."

"I won't."

"God bless you."

"Thanks so much for calling. Bye, Father Justin."

"Bye bye."

My priest told me I can just pray "Lord have mercy," so that's what I'm going to do. Good thing God doesn't require any more, because I don't have it to give.

I return to Little House on the Prairie. I sit through the episode.

And another.

And another.

The rays of sun are lowering.

"Wanna go for a walk?" says Mom. She's long since finished vacuuming and is probably starting to think about dinner.

It was a long and torturous afternoon, and I can hardly believe it's coming to a close.

"Yes."

It's better to be outside where the breeze is, where Mom's attention is on me and not on talking on the phone or cleaning the house or sprouts or kale or the animals.

"Your dad will be home at eight if you can wait till then to have dinner." She likes to call my stepdad "your dad."

"Okay, I don't care when I eat."

The sand is almost hot on my feet, but the air doesn't feel too bad, given it's almost seven. Outside the gate, we turn left. Mom puts both her hands around my left elbow. The evening air and Mom's compassion are warm on my cold heart.

Mom's plan for me being better by the end of the week has failed, and I need to know something now.

"Mom, will you get tired of being here for me?"

"No, never, Honey. I'll *always* be here for you." Gray hair strands sweep the side of her face as she answers.

"What if I don't heal? Will you still sit outside with me at night?"

"Yes I will, but you *will* heal."

"How can you say that?"

"Because I just know."

"But if I don't heal, then I'm afraid you will be disappointed in me."

"Honey, I will *never* be disappointed in you."

"Then why haven't I healed yet?"

"You will heal, but maybe you just aren't going to heal *yet*."

"I'm a failure. All I do is cost you guys money."

"You're here to recover, that's all."

We are at the end of the block, and we turn left.

"I let everyone down and have nothing to give."

"You haven't let anyone down. Someday you'll be able to help others."

"If I heal. I don't know if I'll heal."

"But you will."

The street veers upward, and wind is pushing against us. My muscles strain to take each step. With the setting sun and Mom beside me, I'm numb against the despair, as I was 24 hours ago. I treasure these precious few moments of feeling nothing at all.

5 We could send her in a helicopter

Nine days, no sleep.

My stepdad is here, so it must still be early. It's Saturday, but he often works Saturdays. In the kitchen, Mom is telling him all the things she's putting on his sandwich.

"Sounds good," he says.

I have no sense of it being a Saturday. The only thing different about today is I won't be going to the holistic clinic. This means a longer stretch of morning and an earlier walk.

This bed is a miserable place to be, and being out of it is no more inviting.

I'm not sure what will come out of my mouth when I get up. I need Mom to know I can't keep living. I can't hold that in any longer. But I'll wait till my stepdad is gone before I get out of this bed and start talking.

"When do you think you'll be home?" Mom says.

"Bout eight, I s'pose."

"Okay, I love you so much, Sweetie. See you at eight."

"You, too."

The pounding of his footsteps and the swishing of his slacks and dress shirt pass the hallway entrance and enter the foyer.

"Bye Misty and Tiny," he coos. He's as bad as Mom when it comes to the animals. "Bye bye, Fuzzy. See you later, Nut Nut. Have a good day, Zoom Zoom. You, too, Snowball."

When his Mustang starts, I sit up. I may as well have been run over by a truck. No, not a truck. A *semi*. Maybe a train. I don't even want a shower. I reach for my hair band on my dresser and pull my hair into a low pony tail. I'm in my Hanes outfit from yesterday. All I need are my flip flops, which are on the floor next to my bed.

I'll let Mom make my bed. I need to get out of this house and into the cool morning air as soon as possible because it's the closest I can come to a sense of escape.

I stop in the kitchen to tell Mom I didn't sleep again.

"Oh, *no*," she says. She's scraping wet cat food onto a dish.

I'll get out of here just before feeding time. "Mom, I need to be outside. I'm going for a long walk. Don't worry about me," I say.

"Okay, Honey. Well, later today we'll do some grocery shopping. How does that sound?"

"Whatever, it doesn't matter."

I'm on the road to the park, and on the left is the sand leading to the concrete wall. My head is swelling as if all its molecules are filled to the brim, like always inhaling but never exhaling. I've been expecting an explosion, a tipping point of some sort. The explosion never comes.

Moving my limbs isn't bringing mental relief.

I need relief.

Relief.

What could give me relief? There has to be something.

Something cutting edge, perhaps, and maybe I can hold out till it's discovered.

Then there are drugs. I never want drugs in my body again. My brain was torched on the Klonopin, and now I'm sure it's even more fried from the sleeplessness and less responsive to drugs than ever. Not even a heavy dose of a benzo would touch me now—never mind the myriad of weaker drugs.

"Don't let anyone convince you that you need drugs," the woman from the forum wrote.

I am going to remember that.

That wave of despair is hitting with more intensity, more frequency. That head explosion is *bound* to happen. The repetition of my thoughts is like the circle on this grassy knoll, and I'm going round and round. There's no escape. I think of Mom back home on the phone making raw food and of me at the kitchen table pushing away dogs and cats and watching Little House on the Prairie, and I know I must keep walking on this grass as long as I can.

It's been about an hour and a half, and there's Mom in the Yukon, driving towards me.

Why in the world is she here? She better not be worried about me. She pulls up in front of the park and sticks her head out the window.

I start walking toward her. "Mom, what are you doing here?"

"I'm ready to go grocery shopping. Let's go."

"But I'm not done walking yet."

"We need to go now so that we're home in two hours for me to let the dogs widdle."

"Oh, my gosh."

I walk over and climb into the Yukon.

It's only early afternoon now and we're back in our usual

143

places in the kitchen: Mom at the counter and me on the dining room chair.

"Oh. My. Gosh. *Audrey*. Those oat groats *didn't sprout*."

"Okay."

"They're not *raw!* If they don't sprout, they're *not raw!*"

"Okay, Mom."

The phone rings. It's Granddaddy again, and I cannot fathom this conversation going anywhere productive.

"No, no sleep. Nine days, no sleep," Mom reports to him.

Tension is swelling up in my head.

"Daddy, she's been to doctors back in Kentucky..."

If I hear as many as two more statements about my condition, I'm leaving the room.

"Yes, let's do that. Let's do a conference call."

A what?

"We'll get you, Robbie, Pam and Lisa on the line."

Uncle Robbie, *too?* This can't be.

"Yes, Hi, Lisa. Audrey hasn't slept at all in nine days. I've got Daddy on the line, and he thinks we should do a conference call. Let's see if we can get Pam and Robbie. I'm dialing Pam right now... Pam? We're gonna do a conference call with me, you, Lisa, Robbie, and Daddy about Audrey. Oh... okay... You can do four o'clock your time? You'll call Robbie and tell him? Good. Talk to you in an hour and a half."

She hangs up.

My heart's beating fast, and I get all my energy ready to launch. I will protest this conference call with everything in me.

"Mom, no! Do *not* have a conference call! *Please stop talking* about me! There's nothing you all can do!"

"Audrey, we're just gonna brainstorm, that's all."

"You don't even believe I'm gonna *heal* any more, do you?"

"Yes, I *do* believe you will heal."

"Then why are you doing this? You're just trying to appease *Granddaddy!*"

"Audrey, we are just gonna put our heads together. Just *let* us put our heads together."

"There is *no help* for me! I have *tried* to tell you that, but you won't listen!"

"Audrey, they just wanna help. We're gonna discuss *options.*"

"I *told* you the colon cleansing stuff wasn't gonna help, but you wouldn't listen! Now you don't even think I'm gonna *heal* anymore!"

"I *do* think you're gonna heal!"

"Please don't talk about me! You are all making it worse!"

"We're *just. Gonna. Discuss. Options."*

"There *are* no options! Do you think I haven't tried *everything?* There's not a doctor in the *world* that can help me!"

"Audrey, we're just gonna talk. Now, why don't I make ya a nice salad? I've got nuts, avocados, raisins, olives..."

I'm whimpering. I exerted way too much energy and just elevated my own desperate misery.

I absolutely can't bear to hear myself talked about.

Even by me.

"Daddy? Robbie? Pam and Lisa? Oh, great, I got you all on. Thank you so much. Listen, this week..."

I put my hands over my ears and head straight to the bedroom. I *need* to not hear. I sit on the floor; I don't want to sit on a bed in the middle of the day.

146

"Lalalala, lalalala, lalalala," I repeat with my hands over my ears. I don't know how long this conversation's going to last.

The "lalala's" are taking too much effort. I start humming instead. I pause to see if she's still on the phone.

"Mayo Clinic. Yes, we could fly her there."

I clamp my hands on my ears quick. "Lalalala, lalalala, lalalala."

What a *joke!* What can any doctor in the world do but give me drugs I've already tried? Not to mention that any given doctor is unlikely to be aware of benzo withdrawal.

I loosen my hands from my ears.

"No, the colon cleansing and raw food haven't helped so far, but I'm still hopeful."

"Lalalala. Lalalala."

Mom says she thinks I will heal, but she is just pacifying me. Truth is that she feels helpless. If she didn't, she wouldn't be having this conversation.

I loosen my hands.

"Yeah, we could send her in a helicopter."

I slam my hands hard over my ears. Fury travels through my veins like a current, and my heart jumps at the vision of myself in a helicopter. I can't hear any more of this. I will

147

wait several minutes this time before checking.

Finally, I hear Mom shouting to the dogs that it's time for a treat. I take my hands off my ears and walk out of the bedroom into the kitchen.

"Mayo Clinic?"

"Yes, Honey, that's what we came up with."

The idea of being in any clinic at all—the sterile smell, white walls, and bed tables with paper sheets—is repugnant. Mom is clearing the kitchen counters and not even looking at me.

"I'm *not* going! They can't help me! *No one* can help me! Even the most knowledgeable doctor in the *world* can't help me! There is nothing anyone can do! Why don't you *believe me?"*

I'm exerting the very energy I've been using to guard the hell behind my skin. Now that hell is free to roam, and who knows how much memento it will pick up. I know this, but I don't care. Nothing matters more than putting a stop to their idea of subjecting me to a helicopter and a hospital.

"Honey, we've decided to fly you there as a last resort."

"You guys are *totally* ignorant! I will never go, and you can't force me! You don't *believe* me when I tell you no one can help me!"

Mom closes the cabinet over the olive oil she has just put away and faces me with her hands on her hips.

148

"Audrey, you hafta let me look into this *for myself.* I'm taking care of *you,* and now you let *me* look for answers."

"There *are no* answers! There's no cure for benzo withdrawal except *time!* If benzo withdrawal is even what I *have!*"

"Now, Audrey, I need to look into this for *myself.*"

"You're making everything worse! I can't stand you all talking about me! I can't take it! I *won't* take it! I can die *right here in this house!*"

Mom's lips tighten. She turns away from me and takes a rag to wipe the counters. Her arms jerk in circular motions.

She's angry. Good thing my stepdad's not here.

I slide down and sit Indian style on the ground against the kitchen wall and put my hands over my face. I'm heaving and sobbing though there isn't stamina for it. I am utterly drained from the yelling and have no reserve to draw from; I don't know how my body will withstand this heaving. Poor Mom is angry and I don't blame her, but I can't help myself. The despair is ringing out my soul and body like wet rags, and my wails are thrusting forward with involuntary momentum.

I know this is too much for Mom. But I have no one else to turn to—no one else to listen to me declare my need to die. She is my only audience. My crying is lowering in volume to moderate wails, but I can't achieve the calm that tears are meant to bring forth. My nerves are smoking like sparklers, and nothing can stop the burning.

149

"Mom. I really need you to understand that I can't go on. I can't do this."

She says nothing but her jaw is still clenched as she wipes the counters.

My breaths are short. My wails are dying but there's no relief. I'm silent now and don't know what to do with these quieter moments. I can't begin to stretch my mind around passing the time until evening.

I spent the afternoon in my bedroom on the benzo withdrawal forum telling them about the family conference call, holding my head with my right hand when I wasn't using it to type.

Two of the responses in particular spoke to me, and I keep rereading them. A woman in her fifties with an avatar of herself with large sunglasses and thick salt and pepper hair writes,

"I'm in withdrawal from benzos for the second time. I healed after the first time, and you will, too. The sleep comes back, trust me. It came back for me, and it will for you. You are much younger than me, so your body will heal with no problem. Just don't let anybody, and I mean *anybody,* tell you that you need drugs. That's what happened to me, and now here I am in withdrawal for the second time. First time was five years ago."

Another woman's avatar shows she's a thin brunette, maybe in her forties.

"The brain can start to heal when you stay away from drugs. Many people keep taking new drugs, and it just prolongs the recovery. When you leave your brain alone, it can start to return to normal. Many family members and friends don't understand that and will keep trying to get you back on drugs."

I'm reading their words for the fourth time now. I know they're right. And yet I need their reminders. I'm surrounded by a world that can't be trusted. Family, friends, doctors—they are *all* wrong; they think a drug can work for me, that the right doctor can help me. They think conventional medicine is the answer and that I'm too stubborn to try it. I have tried it numerous times, and all they can think is that I haven't tried it enough. No one wants to believe there's no help for me—it's too awful to believe.

But it's the truth.

It's almost eight p.m. The dogs are bounding toward the front windows and barking wildly because the Mustang is at the gate. Since the dogs are already inside, my stepdad opens the gate himself and closes it after driving through. The front door opens, and here he is with his dress clothes and briefcase and sunglasses resting on top of his head.

I'm standing in the entrance to the kitchen, holding my laptop and trying to decide whether to sit at the kitchen table or retreat to my room. I'm astounded I made it through this day, and it's a good thing he wasn't here for it; he wouldn't

151

have tolerated my fight with Mom. He's too protective of her.

"Well, hi there Zoom Zoom, Fuzzy, Tiny, Misty, Nut Nut."

He walks up and kisses my forehead.

"Hi," I say.

"Hi there, Sweetie. How was your day?"

"Ha."

"What's that supposed to mean?" he says. He's glancing into the kitchen at Mom.

Her lips are still a little tight.

"It was a horrible, horrible day," I say.

"No sleep?"

"No, no sleep," I reply.

He leans forward and gives me a big, long hug. He understands that there aren't any words that can make things better.

He crosses into the kitchen and hugs and kisses Mom. I head over to the kitchen table and sit down.

"Honey!" she says to him, her mood instantly lighter. "Guess what's for dinner? Raw spaghetti!"

"Oh, that sounds fantastic," he says.

His presence has a way of diffusing tension. The lingering words from this afternoon's conversations are evaporating. He puts his briefcase on the couch.

"How was your day, Honey?" asks Mom.

"Well, it was a *day,*" he chuckles, shaking his head.

"Okay, guys, I've got some spaghetti marinara that is *so* good, you won't believe it. Here, Sweetie, sit down next to Audrey. It's ready. Let me just dish it out."

He joins me at the table.

"So, no sleep, huh Augrit?" he says.

"No, none for nine days. Do you think my sleep will come back?" I ask him

"Why, yes, I do," he says.

"Are you just saying that, or do you really think it will?"

"I really think it will," he says.

"How long do you think it will take?" I say.

"Oh, I don't know the answer to that, Sweetie. It's just gonna take some time."

Barbara's voice in my head echoes, *You'll be feeling a lot better by Christmas.*

"Do you think it could be back by Christmas?"

He tilts his head and gives the same chuckle he did when Mom asked him about his day.

"I think you'll *still* be dealing with this at Christmas."

Me, too.

Mom is pulling a large plate out of the dehydrator; it holds zucchini pieces shaped like spaghetti noodles. She divides it into three portions, slides two of them onto smaller plates, and pours the sauce over all three. She dips her finger into the sauce on her plate. *"Mmmmmm."* She smacks her lips. "Lemme tell you what's in this." She looks at us and starts in on the hand motions. "First, I spiralized some zucchini using my spiralizer, as you can see here." She gestures to a white plastic appliance with a crank. "Then, in the blender, I put six fresh Roma tomatoes, raw garlic cloves, olive oil, some dates, fresh basil and oregano, and fresh-squeezed lemon juice. You aren't gonna *believe* it."

"Sounds good, Mom."

She carries two plates to us, walks back to pick up her own, then joins us.

"Mom, can you push Cuddles off the table? His cat hair is disgusting and all over the place."

"Cuddles, let's get down. Get down, now." She nudges him

until he wakes up and leaps to the ground.

The raw "pasta" is warm from the dehydrator. The temperature is just right, really. Not hot, but not entirely cold. The spices have a lot of flavor. It's rich because of the olive oil, I'm sure. The sweetness must be from the dates. This is almost as good as the raw lasagna.

I scarf it down. The momentary sensation on my taste buds is a welcomed distraction.

"Thanks, Mom. That was really good."

Finished with his meal, my stepdad retires to his place on the far right of the green couch.

I sit on the other side of it for a change of scenery from the kitchen chair. The floor lamp illumines the forest green fabric and makes it look soft.

Zoom Zoom jumps up next to me and is nestling his snout into my sides. I push him off and hold my bended legs up to my knees to communicate I don't want company. But he keeps pressing his snout on me. I slap his snout, and he sits up straight and paws my arm. Like a deranged Coyote, he's looking past me rather than at me.

"Will someone *please* get him off me?"

"Zoom Zoom, down. Leave Audrey alone," Mom calls.

Zoom Zoom leaps down and trots away. Three other dogs are sprawled on the floor. Dinky is perched behind me on the couch back, her usual position; Snowball is resting on the kitchen counter behind me, his stomach pooling out in all directions; Cuddles is on the cat bed by the television. Peanut is nestled in Pumpkin's torso between me and my stepdad.

Mom wants to know all about his day, shooting twenty questions from the kitchen while he's trying to answer emails.

"Mom, he doesn't like being bombarded with questions when he's trying to answer emails. Don't you get that?"

"Oh, Honey, he *loves* it when I ask him questions. Don't you?" She smiles at the back of his head.

Not looking up from his laptop, he half-grins and says, "Why, yes, I love it."

The seconds don't seem to pass. Maybe talking will help.

"So, how was your day?" I ask him.

"It was just alright. Had to fire someone."

"Oh," I say. "How did you do it?"

"Told him I had to let him go. He doesn't show up to work and then gets an attitude every time I give him a warning."

"Oh, gotcha... Um, are you *sure* you think I'm gonna get better?"

"Yes." He looks up at me from his laptop for just a moment.

156

"You're not just saying that?"

"No, not just sayin' it, Honey."

"Lots of people in benzo withdrawal get better in six months. Six months from now is Christmas. But you don't think I'll be better by Christmas?"

He chuckles again and shakes his head.

"Like I said, I think you'll still be dealing with this at Christmas."

"But you think I will get better someday?"

"Yes."

His "s" has a little lisp, and the stubble on his chin is shining in the lamplight.

6 A blue hue of moonlight

March 1989 LaPorte, Indiana

Todd was family.

An unspoken pact occurred in our huddle on the snow. I would do nothing more to ruin his life with us at The Back Nine. At night, I darted upstairs early to my bedroom so I wouldn't have to stand there while everyone else said they loved him.

Todd brought old photos of himself from Goldy's. Back home, he set them on our dining room table.

I kept returning to them.

I held these photos after school while sitting on the dining room chair by the sliding wood door. Forgetting a sense of time, I gazed at the young Todd. The pictures told me Todd was more than the wiry stranger with stringy hair who'd invaded our family.

"These are the only pictures Goldy has of Todd," said Mom.

There were five photos. Three were Todd's grade school pictures: Kindergarten, Second grade, and Fifth grade. He wore the same expression in each: meek and obliging. He smiled at the world beyond the camera as if saying he didn't have much to offer, but what he had, he would give. His shiny dark hair was parted on the side, ending in uneven jags. His mom must have cut his hair when she was still alive. In one school photo, his skinny arms rested on a flat surface. His glasses were the same in all three pictures: chunky, dark frames and lenses half an inch thick.

Another photo showed a five-year-old Todd ripping a piece of wrapping paper off his present on Christmas morning, his right arm flying back. Mom stood behind my shoulder as we looked at Todd's excited face.

"That would have been the only present Todd got that Christmas," she said. "He often got no presents at all. Todd didn't have toys."

So *that* was why Todd got so lost in playing with Kelsey's toys.

The last picture was Todd at age three. Small as he was, he wore the same thick glasses. A diaper bulged under his cotton pants, giving the only appearance of mass on his spindly body.

"Mommy, why is Todd wearing glasses in this picture?"

"His mom was a drug addict. She let him crawl around the

house all by himself. When he was two years old, he bit into an electrical cord—the cord of a fan. He got electrocuted and that's why his eyes are crossed. It's just so *sad.*" Tears poured from her eyes and she nodded.

I was sad too. The sadness was like a bubble in my heart that got bigger and bigger as I looked at the pictures. I thought the bubble would burst and that I would start to cry. But I didn't.

I imagined little Todd moving inside the still pictures then crawling toward the electrical cord and biting it.

I shuddered.

I watched him tear open his only gift at Christmas. I wished he had more gifts to open. But he was so happy with just the one. I saw him pose for his school pictures, then lift himself off the stool and walk down the school hall. Did he have any friends at school? Did he get any love when he got home?

I had a sinking feeling when I thought about his childhood.

I was very, very glad Todd now had toys to play with. And a family at The Back Nine that loved him.

I started being extra nice to him.

June 2009 Clove Valley, CA

I'm back in my bedroom—I told Mom I was getting into bed, careful not to say the word "sleep." I won't let Mom and my stepdad forget my suffering. I want to be alone tonight. I don't want to touch Mom, let alone hold onto her, after her call with Lisa, Pam, Robbie and Granddaddy. They're just like everybody else, and even Mom has turned on me. There is now no one that can understand but the members of the forum.

Mayo Clinic. Truly unbelievable.

I discovered on the park bench that November day back in Kentucky that benzo withdrawal was the best bet for what I had, but I wouldn't tell Dr. Hoback that. I couldn't bear the thought of opening up, making myself vulnerable to his disbelief, his condescension. He'd told me I could discontinue Klonopin abruptly. He hadn't mentioned withdrawal, so he wouldn't believe me if I told him what the drug had done to me.

And I *needed* something from him: one final prescription for a five-month taper at 5% weekly reduction. I couldn't take a chance of rocking the boat.

Thankfully, he wrote the final prescription, with slight exasperation behind his eyes as I explained I'd decided to get off Klonopin slowly.

I didn't tell him I'd obtained one type of sleeping pill after another from the emergency clinic in hopes of finding a magic drug to replace Klonopin. I didn't tell him the herbs, vitamins, minerals, salts, and other remedies I'd tried. I didn't tell him I'd taken Doxepin with two alcoholic drinks, still unable to pass out. I didn't tell him I'd thrown my bottle of Klonopin in the Dumpster outside my apartment and, after 48 hours of no sleep, climbed in it and turned over trash till I spotted the bottle with 14 pills remaining.

He didn't need to know any of that. No one else needed to know either. The world had become unsafe—a place where no help can be found, where lives are destroyed by casually prescribed drugs, and where no one takes my word for anything.

And now Mom has the audacity to suggest I'll fly in a helicopter to see a doctor.

I'm climbing under the covers. The glaring daylight is behind me, and the night sky outside the window touches me with coolness, assuring me I'm shielded from people for the next eight hours.

"Mom," I call.

"Yes, Honey," she answers. Her feet pound down the hallway, and she appears in the doorway.

"Will you say a couple of evening prayers for me?"

"Yes, of course." She sits on the end of my bed by my legs.

"Okay, thank you so much, Mom. It won't take long... just maybe the beginning prayers and one evening prayer. I'll show you."

The honeycomb beeswax candles are in a row next to my icon of Christ. I move one forward and light it. The print of His face is illumined by the flame. The folded up messages from forum members promising I'll heal is next to my blue prayer book. I flip to *Prayers Before Sleep*. I hand her the prayer book and pull the covers over me.

"Okay," she says, taking the book.

"Thanks so much, Mom. You have no idea what this means. I don't have the energy to pray, but if you pray then I can listen."

"I'm so glad to. Are you ready?"

"Yes."

She says the *Trisagion Prayers,* or prayers to the Trinity. Then she says the first evening prayer. I am half-listening, thankful that her words are a substitute for mine. The beeswax candle flame is flickering.

She's done, and I say, "Thank you so much, Mom. It helps a lot. Will you say these prayers with me anytime I need you to?"

"Yes, Honey, anytime."

"You won't get tired of praying when I ask you to?"

"No. It's the least I can do."

"Thank you so much, Mom."

"You are so welcome, Honey. I just love you *so* much."

"I love you too, Mom."

"You try to rest tonight, okay?"

"I won't sleep but I will try to feel like I'm resting."

"You never know. Tonight could be the night."

"Sorry for all I'm putting you through. I don't know what I'd do without your help."

"Oh, I'm glad to help. Just *so* glad. I'd do anything to help you, Audrey. If only I could take your place, I would."

"I would never want you to go through this. I'd rather suffer than any of you suffer."

"I'd gladly suffer in your place... if God would just *let* me." Thin tears glide down her cheeks.

"No, Mom, I don't want you to suffer. I just don't want to let you all down."

"You're not letting us down."

"If I don't get better, I will let you all down."

"But you will get better."

"I can't believe that, but thank you for believing it for me."

"I *do* believe it."

"Okay. Thanks for praying for me."

"You gonna go night-night now?"

"I'm ready to lie here in the dark with the lights out."

"Okay, night-night, Sweetie."

She kisses my cheek and turns off the parrot lamp.

"Mom, since no animals can get in here, can I keep the candle burning for a little while?"

"Okay," she says. "That should be okay."

She closes the door behind her.

Laying on my right side, I'm eye level with the dresser. I reach for the icon of Christ and hold it in front of me on the bed. The candle flame lights up the right side of His face.

However remote, He is somehow here. I wonder how well He can hear me. The sleeplessness in my body is thick as steel. Can He get through it? His face in the icon is gentle. With the beeswax candle burning and Mom's prayers settling in the room, the steel in my body seems to soften a little. So does the steel in my soul.

I think He might be hearing me.

Lord, please heal me. I have gone nine days with no sleep. Will you please give me at least a foretaste of healing? Even just five minutes of sleep? If I really am going to heal, will you show me? Give me a tiny glimpse?

I put the icon back on the dresser against the wall and blow out the candle. My cell phone says 9:23 p.m. I lay my head back down on the pillow.

Nine days, no sleep. One of these nights, something might be different. The ability to drift off, though it's been lost, could come back. The impossible might become possible. I don't know when that time will come.

I close my eyes and feel drowsy, knowing drowsiness no longer has a connection to sleep. But I still hope my mind will drift off.

I awaken.

Awaken?

I slept. I really just slept. That old feeling of waking up from a deep sleep is here, for the first time in nine days. I'm dying to know how long. I grab my cell phone.

It's 9:53 p.m. I slept for 30 minutes.

It's the foretaste!

Five minutes, or even three, would have been a foretaste. But

166

I got *30*. My body has the ability to fall asleep!

A blue hue of moonlight through the curtains illumines His face on the dresser.

He heard me.

Mom drives away in the Yukon, leaving me at the Orthodox Church in La Joleta. The sun through the stained glass windows can't wash this place out because the walls are already stark white. The icon greeting me inside the door is an older and faded print of The Ladder of Divine Ascent. I cross myself and bow three times while kissing the icon.

Hard to believe I'm doing this. I feel very weak and like an alien inside a body that looks normal. Other than the blissful half an hour of sleep between 9:23 and 9:53 last night, I got none. Not sure what it will be like to sit through the service. But I have to be somewhere, and that place might as well be here.

Around the corner to the left is the nave. The iconostasis in front is the main source of color: rich, bold colors in the clothing of Mary, Christ, angels, saints, and apostles. The pews are sparsely dotted with dark-haired families and some elderly people. The choir is a few out-of-key individuals, including a skinny older man whose voice is shaking in tremors. Up front is the priest with a graying beard and stocky frame. Some are standing and others are sitting. It's only been a few minutes since liturgy started, and I'm trying to stand, but my stamina's run out.

I take a seat. Sitting is more tolerable, though trying to pay attention to the words strains my mind.

It's time to take communion. I get in line behind the fifteen or so others going up. The priest asks my name.

"Audrey. My saint name is Sophia."

He places the spoon in my mouth. I swallow the bread and wine and veer to the left behind the others. I stop at the corner in front of an icon of Mary holding Christ.

Their faces are smooth and life-like. As I look into her eyes I'm feeling her presence like I felt I felt the presence of Christ last night. She is near, not far, and she's listening.

"Please," I whisper. "Please ask your son Jesus to heal me."

There's a tray of thin beeswax candles on the table below the icon. I light one from the flame in the gold candle holder and stick it in the sandbox with the others. I return to my pew; the service is almost over. It's time to go up and kiss the cross the priest is holding.

"You are welcome to join us for a meal after the service," he says as I lift my face from the cross.

"Okay, thank you. I will."

Back in the foyer and to the left, a wide open room has folding tables and chairs; the table up front is holding cheese slices, bagels and fruit. I put some fruit on a plate and sit at the table closest to the foyer where a middle-aged woman is seated. She looks up at me as I sit down.

"Hi, I'm Sarah."

"Hi, nice to meet you. I'm Audrey."

"Do you live in La Joleta?"

"Well, no, I live in Kentucky, but I'm here with my mom and stepdad due to a health issue."

"Oh, I see. Well, do you think you might recover sometime soon?"

"I don't know if I will. I could be here long term."

"I see. The priest will have to pray for you, then. You should ask him."

"Thank you. I was planning to ask if I could meet with him for holy unction."

"You can. Do let him know. He would be happy to pray for you. We do have coffee. Would you like some?"

"Oh... No, thank you. I avoid caffeine. I was on a large tranquilizer and built up tolerance to it and had to get off. Now I cannot sleep at all."

"Oh, I *know* what that's like. I've been there. I couldn't sleep about five years ago. The doctor gave me Ambien, and now I can sleep."

"So you do know what it's like. I had to increase my dose because it quit working. Then the larger dose stopped working well, too. Now no doctor would give me the amount needed to put me to sleep."

"I take the same dose he gave me five years ago. It's always worked the same."

"You are really lucky," I say. "Some people build up tolerance."

"Well, now I'm worried."

"Oh, don't be worried... if you've been on the same amount that long and it still works, then you will probably be fine."

"My son had the same thing... he couldn't sleep. He has health issues and the pain kept him awake. He got on Ambien, too."

The stuff seems to put a lot of other people to sleep, but it sure didn't touch me.

"I've tried everything and nothing has worked," I say. "I just have to wait and see if my sleep will come back."

"Oh, but not sleeping is *dangerous,*" she says.

Thanks for the reminder.

"I really don't have any other option. I was on the largest amount most doctors would give, and it was only a matter of time till it quit working. I had no choice but to get off it."

"Have you thought about going back to the doctor?"

"I've gone to lots of doctors. I've already tried all the other drugs for sleep and they didn't work."

"Well, I'm *worried* about you. I know what it's like to just lie there and lie there and not be able to go to sleep."

Yeah. Me, too.

"I'm worried about myself, too, but there's just nothing any doctor can do."

"You might want to give some of those drugs another try."

"I can think about it."

"Yes, I hope you will."

I've just been punched and my soul is dizzy. "My mom is probably here, so I better get going. It was nice to meet you."

"Very nice to meet you, too. Hope you'll come back."

"I'll be back."

"Let the priest know you'd like him to pray for you."

"I will. I'll be giving him a call soon."

Back through the foyer and outside the door is Mom in the Yukon with her nose in a book. I climb in and grip the handle. It's after 12 and warming up. The moments of divine

171

providence visited on me last night have been clawed aside like spider webs. Sarah thinks I'm negligent. She thinks I should go to a doctor and get back on drugs.

Just don't let anybody, and I mean anybody, tell you that you need drugs, said the woman from the forum.

Mom puts the Yukon in drive. "How was church, Honey?"

"It was okay. It's good that I took communion."

"Oh, good. Did you meet anyone?"

"Just a woman during coffee hour. She thinks I should try to get back on drugs that I already know don't work."

Heavy despair is squeezing all my insides, and tears begin to stream. That I'm fighting to stay alive wasn't enough for Sarah. I'm in a sinking sand of shame.

"Mom, it's like people think I'm failing to do something. They don't understand that there's no help for me in drugs."

After yesterday's conference call, she might very well be one of those people. But I'm still going to state the truth until she sees it.

"I know, Honey, I know."

7 Showin' how funky and strong is your fight

June 2009 Two weeks later

I am getting an average of half an hour sleep each night now. Some nights 45 minutes, some an hour and a half, some none. It's hard to celebrate those little bits when my body has a sleep deficit the size of Texas. I still expect physical deterioration or a psychological implosion to happen.

Mom hasn't mentioned Mayo Clinic again, and the conference call was two weeks ago from yesterday. She must have figured it made more sense to take me to doctors in Clove Valley first. So we went to two, and not with my consent.

My need for relief and my lack of caring one way or the other led me to do what the forum members said *not* to: take drugs.

It's said that insanity is doing the same thing over and over expecting a different result, and I thought: *maybe I can try these drugs again with the result of getting some sleep.*

Ten days ago Mom took me to the first doctor. In the waiting room, the misery was like the California heat, baking me outside and in, tormenting me so much that it seemed my life could not possibly be real. In the doctor's office, hearing Mom talk about me to the doctor was even worse than hearing her talk about me to Granddaddy. Add to that the doctor's puzzled facial expression, and there was no place on earth more awful.

"It's like this drug Klonopin just *ruined her life!"* Mom concluded to him.

It was like being sick in the stomach and *then* getting punched. The truth as she saw it came out—she didn't think I'd heal after all. She confirmed what I felt in every sinew of my body.

He prescribed me Seroquel, an anti-psychotic I'd tried once already.

"It didn't put me to sleep in the past, but maybe it will now," I said.

"Yes, it will," he said.

We got home from the pharmacy, and Mom suggested I take the Seroquel right away.

"Maybe you'll get a nice nap," she said.

I doubted it, but the possibility of relief made me give in, and I decided to get it over with. I took it and lay down on the floor of my stepdad's sports room, where collectable sports figures in their original packaging are nailed up high all around the room where the walls meet the ceiling, and a glass case of shotguns sits against a set of sliding glass patio doors.

The rays of sun through the glass doors created a smog effect, and I began to feel strange, drowsy, and disoriented. The shotguns stared at me from their case. I achieved nothing close to sleep and got up from the mattress after two hours to be near Mom on the living room couch.

Two days later I was in the second doctor's office.

Mom asked the doctor questions, trying to find out what might be wrong with me. I jumped in and said the Klonopin had done this and that no one could help me. The doctor said he'd never heard of a condition like mine and referred me to a sleep clinic. When Mom looked hopeful and asked what a sleep clinic could do, I yelled that a sleep clinic could do nothing. I ran out of the office and into the parking lot.

I found a grassy knoll beside the parking lot and sobbed. Mom came out of the office ten minutes later and headed for the Yukon. I went toward the Yukon and said, "I told you not to do this to me!"

A family getting out of their car stared. Mom's lips were totally tightened down as she climbed in and started the Yukon.

"You have no idea, *no idea* what you just did! I can *barely survive,* and you take me to the worst place on earth I could be—a *doctor's office!"*

My insides ran a marathon, and my chest was heaving as I got in on the passenger's side. But that wasn't going to stop me.

Mom's face was full of fury and her hands were on the steering wheel so tight that they were red.

"You want a *second opinion.* You think the doctor knows something I don't. I told you a doctor can't help. But you *wouldn't believe me!"*

We pulled out of the parking lot and took some turns and were back on a main road. Then Mom pulled over. She turned to me with hot tears on her red face.

"You listen *here.* You are killing me—*killing me!* I have aged *ten years* since you got here. You cannot live with me and do this to me—you're gonna send me to my grave! I have the *right* to look for answers. I have the *right* to get a second opinion."

My insides were raked by my yelling and filled with shock at hers. I imagined her face looking older than when I first got to Clove Valley. My wails became whimpers; I needed to quiet down fast. Mom put her head on the steering wheel and sobbed. I didn't dare say anything for two minutes.

Then I said, "Mom, you can look for answers; just don't take me with you."

She lifted her tear-soaked face back up and said, "You cannot, *cannot,* keep doing this to me!"

"I won't, Mom, I won't! I promise! I appreciate everything you are doing. As long as I never have to go to the doctor again, I will be good, I promise!"

"I will *not* let you ruin my life!"

"I won't! I'll keep my thoughts to myself! Just don't take me to the doctor, that's *all I ask!*"

"If you're gonna scream at me like you did in that parking lot, you *can't* live here," she said.

"Feel free to send me to an insane asylum. It's where I belong anyway!" I said.

"I've aged *ten years,* and you will *not* do this to me!"

"Okay!"

We got home.

I didn't imagine my existence had a purpose. But it did. For all the things I couldn't do, there was one thing I could do. I could try to be nice to Mom.

I could say thank you more often. I could put up less of a fight when she asked me to load dishes and do other chores. I could stop making threats.

I could stop aging her.

177

Today is Sunday. I didn't go to liturgy last weekend, and I don't have the motivation to go this morning. Plus Sarah's words left a bad taste in my mouth.

"Audrey, it looks like we're gonna get transferred soon," says Mom. "Your dad is gonna find out soon where the company is moving us."

"How soon?"

"Within the next couple months."

Ha. A couple of *months*.

I won't be here by then.

"Any idea where?"

"Not yet. We're hoping for somewhere in the Midwest though. Can you help me load these dishes?"

Fury shoots through me. I'm at my usual spot at the kitchen table with my hand covering my face.

"Mom, I need to sit here. Just trust me. I need to sit here."

"Just do some dishes. It'll be a good distraction."

"No, Mom, no. Please believe me. It's taking everything in me just to stay alive right now. I can't move."

Her lips are ever so slightly tightening. Her limbs are jerking just a little.

178

"I *really* need your help."

No, she really doesn't.

"Mom, you don't understand. I'm using all the energy I have to try and stay alive. Please believe me."

"Just try it," she says. "I think you'll be surprised."

"Oh, my gosh."

I really do need to stay at this table and hold the hell inside my skin. But I get up, remembering I can make her life a little more bearable if I do. I let tears fall so Mom sees my face and doesn't forget my suffering.

She's washing off dishes and handing them to me. I'm bending down and loading each one into the dishwasher.

The repetitive bending motion is actually a little distracting.

This isn't so bad.

April 1989 LaPorte, Indiana

Spring came. Heavy raindrops fell in large pelts that ruptured the surface of the lake and streams. The rain was so heavy it billowed like sheets. The world as I knew it was getting a warm bath, and we'd stop and watch through the living room windows. Whoever was in charge of the world must have some kind of joy—He was suspending everything and giving us all a recess. A break from thoughts of ugly neighborhoods and houses with junk that never got thrown out; little kids who got electrocuted and cross-eyed because their moms didn't take care of them.

When the rain stopped, I went outside and smelled the dew on the grass. The sunshine and spring breezes had the feel of magic. The property was alive.

On a Spring night, Todd went to look for our missing dog Buster while Mom, Della, Kelsey and I waited in the room of our house that Mom used for an office. The room had a desk, a computer, and windows that showed the gravel driveway to the gate. Kelsey and Della, four and six years old, sat on the floor hugging their knees under a mirror framed with white-painted wood. We'd been crying steadily since noticing Buster had disappeared.

Todd opened the front door and leaned halfway in to tell us the news. "I've got him," he said, tears on his face—the second time I saw him cry. "He's in the back of the Suburban."

Todd went to retrieve a tarp from the barn to cover Buster's body for the night. Mom told us he'd bury Buster in the morning. Death wafted over the back of the Suburban a few yards outside our front door. The office shielded us from it, though not quite enough.

Several minutes later, Todd rejoined us. He told us how it happened.

"Buster got out of the fence to visit his friend and got hit."

We knew Buster escaped each week to visit his dog friend. This time, though, he wasn't coming back.

We were shocked.

Buster and his brother Chuck were a few months older than me. I'd seen photographs of me as an infant leaning in the grass onto Buster's snout, gripping his ears. Buster came with us when we moved to Indiana and Chuck stayed with my dad.

Up until Buster died, I had daydreamed about him from my school desk, wondering if his water bowl was dry back home. What if he had knocked it over and spilled it? If he had... his mouth might be dry for hours till I could refill it. Unless he had been smart enough to go down to the creek and lap some water. I'd hoped he was that smart. I had told Buster I loved him when I petted him, but he had looked kind of oblivious. I had worried whether he understood me and knew he was loved.

As he lay in the back of the Suburban, I worried again. What if he didn't know I loved him? He would be even more unable to know, now that he lay still with no breath in him.

"Buster was a *good* dog," Mom wailed and nodded in the office chair wearing a long-sleeved black Danskin and grey sweatpants. Her mascara streaks matched her Danskin, and her dark wavy hair was barely lighter. She wiped her face with a tissue and nestled her bare feet into the carpet.

181

Kelsey, his shaved head buried in his knees, started a new round of sobs.

"He was my favorite dog in the *whole wide world!*" I said, spinning my revolving office chair in slow circles.

Della sobbed steadily, her little stomach jumping up and down. A long stringy strand of brown hair rested on her back—the result of a recent haircut during which the stylist took things into her own hands and gave her a "tail."

Something wasn't right at The Back Nine, where the air that held breezes and warm rain also held a lifeless black Labrador Retriever—the dog I had loved and cared for. What was death, and why was it here? I had a sinking feeling it was here to stay and wouldn't go away for the rest of my life.

Todd walked over and rested his arm on Mom's shoulder.

Our cries began to sputter and die after 45 minutes. I was numb and lethargic from crying. I hoped I didn't hurt poor Buster's feelings when I couldn't generate any more tears. I thought he must be even more sensitive now that he didn't have the benefit of being alive to help ward off emotions. I spun my chair in rapid circles to hide my dry cheeks and listless expression.

In the morning, Todd buried Buster down the hill, across and to the right of all the streams. That afternoon, I asked him to show me Buster's grave. Todd and I walked through sunny breezes to some grass-less earth at the far right of the property. We came up to it, and Todd pointed to an area ted.

"There," he said.

I wondered how close Buster was to the surface of the earth. My stomach churned as I tried to trace his outline with my eyes.

"How deep did you bury him?"

"Hard to say," said Todd. "The hole I dug was 'bout four feet."

"Oh."

Death had moved from the back of the Suburban to a permanent location on The Back Nine. My stomach had a sick feeling. Sometimes I would visit Buster's grave and other times just gaze down at it from the living room window. His body was a ball of dark tucked in the earth, the only thing that kept The Back Nine from being at peace.

What kind of world was this? Death invading life. Something that made me feel sick mixing up with the good things. And death seemed the stronger one.

June 2009 Clove Valley, California

It's afternoon and I'm sitting at a small desk in the living room instead of the kitchen table. I cannot escape my skin and it's too hot to go outside, so I changed my location. I am unbearably agitated, and I'm not sure how to get Mom to understand just how excruciating this is. She's so used to my whining and crying, she probably doesn't think I'm serious when I say I need relief.

So I'm going to use a tone of voice with a whole new level of seriousness.

"Mom... *Mom.*"

"Yes, Honey," she says. She's got sprouts, sunflower seeds, flax seeds, and salt on the kitchen counter and is filling a big glass bowl with water.

"I need relief. I really mean it this time."

"Okay."

Her tone, so far, says she's taking me seriously. Good.

"I know I've said this before. But I really, *really* mean it now. I need *relief.*"

"Okay, I hear ya."

But aside from an anesthetic the size of what just killed Michael Jackson, or enough benzo to sedate an elephant, there's nothing that can knock me out, and we both know that.

There is *something,* though. Something I could get while we are still living in California, before my stepdad gets transferred. I've come across it only rarely in forums and drug reviews. Supposedly, it's not addicting and has helped

184

some people sleep. I seriously doubt it could help me. But, it's unlike anything else I've tried, so I'm curious. I don't know if Mom will go for this—that's why I need her to take me *very* seriously when I say I've reached my limit.

"Mom, you would do anything to help me, right?"

"Like what?"

Here goes.

"Mom, I've read that medical marijuana helps some people sleep in withdrawal. It acts on different brain receptors than other drugs. It's legal here, and I would need to get it soon, before we have to leave to go wherever we're getting transferred."

"Okay. Where can you get some?"

Her tone says she's tense. I'm already prepared; on the laptop screen is a list of doctors in California who prescribe medical marijuana.

"The closest one is an hour away. His fee is $200."

"Okay, well, how do you get in for an appointment?"

The tension in her voice is building, but she's masking it.

"The website says I can call and make an appointment, and I need to bring my birth certificate."

She's stirring the thick mixture of flax seeds, sunflower

seeds, sprouts, and salt in the glass bowl, and her limbs are flinching.

Mom easily spends two hundred dollars on a week's supply of natural groceries. That colon cleansing cost a heck of a lot more than two hundred dollars, too. And she said she'd take my place if God would let her.

But she's not going to take me to get medical marijuana.

"Okay, well, give them a call, I suppose, if this is *really* what you think you need to do."

Those words housed a familiar ticking time bomb.

Mom has moderate agoraphobia, and she doesn't like to leave the dogs and cats by themselves for more than two hours. We'd be on the road for that amount of time *alone,* and that doesn't include the doctor's visit and pick-up of the marijuana.

"I *really do,* Mom. I wouldn't do this if I didn't *absolutely* need relief."

"Okay, then."

"I mean it, Mom. I *really* mean it when I say I need relief."

"I said *okay.*"

"When can we go? I will call to make the appointment. I just need to know when you can take me."

"Well, I don't know. Maybe Thursday."

"Okay. I'll see if I can get in Thursday."

"You know, the animals *really* can't be alone that long."

As I suspected.

"Mom, yes they *can!*"

"You know, two hours in the car and who knows *how* long in this strange town I've never been to, and the dogs are gonna *hafta* widdle."

"Can't you leave the dogs outside? Just while we're gone?"

"Oh, I don't know about *that.*"

"*Moooom!* Are you saying you aren't going to take me? I thought you'd do anything for me! This is the only thing I haven't tried! You said you would do anything for me, but you didn't really *mean* it!"

"This is *out* of my *comfort* zone."

"What *part* is out of your comfort zone? Leaving the dogs?"

"The dogs *can't* be alone that long."

"That's what this is about? The *dogs?*"

"No, it's *not* just about the dogs."

187

"Is it that it's marijuana?"

"I don't *like* it."

"But it's safe! It's not habit forming! It's way safer than that horrible drug I was on!"

She's spreading the seed mixture on dehydrator trays, and her lips are clenched all the way in.

"I'm not *comfortable* with it."

"Mom, I need relief! You aren't willing to do what it takes to give me relief!"

I cry with my face in my hands.

The chance is slim that the marijuana would put me to sleep anyway.

But it was worth a shot.

It's only 6:30 a.m., and there is no way, *no way,* I can make it through this day. My stepdad just walked out the door, and I hear his Mustang start up. When I told Mom yesterday I needed relief, I wasn't exaggerating. By the time this day is over, she'll wish she'd agreed to the marijuana.

The hammer of despair isn't just hitting me every second; it's hitting me every *moment*—dozens of *times* per second. My will to live was shot through completely weeks ago. This morning, I'm infinitely worse than a vegetable.

There is no way I'm making it through this day.

None.

I leave my bedroom and crouch in the corner of the front room with my head in my knees and my arms around my legs.

Zero sleep last night. Not even the half an hour or forty-five minutes that had become possible. My muscles are swelled and I'm trapped inside my body with no escape. My will to stay alive isn't enough to goad me even to take a walk on the grass.

Or enough to motivate me to sign onto the benzo withdrawal forum.

I won't even watch Little House on the Prairie.

I simply *can't* be in this body any longer. I lift my head from my knees just enough to call out. "Mom, Mom. Come here."

She walks in from the kitchen.

"Mom, I can't make it through this day."

"You can't?"

She actually sounds like she's taking me seriously.

189

"No. It's only 6:30 and I don't know how I'll even make it through the next minute."

"Are you sure?"

"I'm sure."

Yesterday's tension is gone from her voice.

"Okay, Honey. Okay. Let me get the dogs fed, and we'll take you somewhere. Is that what you need?"

"Yeah."

"Where do you want to go?"

The place you go when something's really wrong and you want the illusion that something could help.

"I don't know," I say.

"The Emergency Room?" she says.

"Yeah."

"Okay. Okay. We'll get you there. I have to feed the animals and then we'll get you there. Could be about half an hour. You need a shower?"

"No."

Adrenaline is rising in my bloodstream.

190

Adrenaline—that's the *real* reason I am going to the E.R. The fantasy that they can help me is rushing through my veins with an energy of urgency.

We're in the Yukon on the main highway outside our neighborhood. "Mom, I'm sorry. I know this trip is going to cost a lot."

Mom's features are soft. "Honey, don't you worry about that."

"Okay, thank you Mom."

"Here we are."

The emergency room waiting area is some metal chairs pushed up against two walls. Mom gets a clipboard from the lady behind the sliding window and comes back to me. I hold her forearm with both hands as she fills in, on the papers, the answers that she already knows. I'm hunched over so my face isn't visible to the two others waiting.

"Thank you, Mom, for filling this out for me."

"Absolutely, Sweetie."

Mom asks me for the answers she doesn't know and I mutter them. After fifteen minutes, my name is called, and Mom and I follow a male nurse into a cubicle with curtains on all sides. I climb onto the bed and lie back. Mom is in a chair beside me holding my right arm with her hands.

The nurse is clean cut with brown hair and not much older

191

than me.

"Okay, let's see... your paperwork says 'no sleep.'"

"Yeah," I say, adrenaline pumping full force. "I'm not sure if there's something anyone can do. I get an average of half an hour sleep a night. I got off a heavy dose of Klonopin."

"Hmmm... We're pretty limited here in our ability to prescribe psychiatric drugs given that we're a hospital," he says. "I'll talk with the doctor and see what we can do, but then I'll need to refer you to an outpatient clinic."

Mom's eyes get wide. "Oh?" she says. "Do you know of a good one?"

"Yes, we recommend one twenty minutes from here that does a full psychiatric interview."

Oh, no.

"Oh, yes, that's what we want to do!" Mom says, nodding and smiling as if she won something. "Can you give us directions?"

"Yes, I will. I'll talk to the doctor, and then when I come back I'll explain where it's located. It'll be just a few minutes."

I lie back on the table.

The rush of being in an emergency room cubicle is carrying me afloat, so much so that I can ignore the threat of an impending trip to a psychiatric clinic. Mom looks at me, still nodding. She grips my arm tighter and is frowning in a way that shows she's sorry for my suffering.

The feeling of being loved is mixing into the adrenaline. I don't even have the ability to be mad about what's coming next.

"Mom, will you pray the Lord's prayer with me?"

"Yes, Honey." Her hands leave my arm and grab my two hands. Her sitting and me lying back, I start, and she joins me.

"Our Father, who art in heaven, hallowed be Thy name. Thy Kingdom come, Thy will be done, on earth as it is in heaven. Give us this day our daily bread; and forgive us our debts as we forgive our debtors. And lead us not into temptation, but deliver us from the evil one."

The adrenaline convinces me we're two heroic characters calling for help in the middle of an epic battle. Mom is cooperating like an actor faithfully playing her role. The nurse comes in with a slip of paper and stands at the foot of my table.

"I talked to the doctor, and the most we can give you is one and a half milligrams," he says, handing Mom the prescription.

It's for Klonopin.

"It's not enough to put me to sleep," I say. "But that's okay. I wouldn't take it anyway."

The complete pointlessness of this trip to the E.R. is becoming clear.

"That's as much as we can give you, because we are a hospital and not a psychiatric clinic."

I glance at Mom, who is looking at the nurse with large eyes of expectation.

"That's okay. That's okay. I'm gonna take her to that clinic you mentioned. Can you give us directions?"

I'm being offered a single dose of Klonopin I'd never touch, and Mom is determined to take me to this outpatient clinic. The adrenaline rush has slowed to a trickle, and it's about over.

There is nowhere in the world I want to be less than a psychiatric clinic in the California desert.

Mom looks at the nurse. "I'm gonna take her to this clinic. What we really need to get her on is some Luvox. Do you think they'll be willing to prescribe that?"

Oh, no.

Luvox.

Luvox may as well be magic fairy dust, the way Mom sees it. Kelsey has been on it for Obsessive Compulsive Disorder for fifteen years, and Mom has tried to push it on me anytime I felt down. "It's just an *amazing* drug, Audrey!" she'd say. "Just look how it's helped your brother!" This time, she won't relent; she's been through too much since I came home. She'll hand me the pill and watch till I put it in my mouth. I'll have to pretend to swallow it.

This trip to the E.R. has really, *really* backfired.

"They'll do a full evaluation of her symptoms. As to what they will prescribe, I can't be sure, but they will prescribe whatever drugs they think will treat her condition."

"Oh, *fantastic*." Mom looks at me and nods as if I'm excited too. "This is great." She looks back at the nurse. "Can you explain how to get there?"

He's gesturing toward the highway and telling her the two main roads that lead to the clinic. It's about a 20-minute drive.

We are on the road again. Hope has been thoroughly sucked out of every molecule in me as if with a wet-dry vacuum. I'm moaning and whimpering but I don't dare yell. We arrive at the one-story brick clinic. It's surrounded by empty desert terrain except for a hill of huge rocks that border it on one side.

We go in together and Mom goes up to the front desk. The large waiting room to the right has a couple rows of black chairs. I'm the only one here except a janitor vacuuming the maroon carpet and a thin teenage guy on his cell phone explaining that he was brought here after being arrested for public intoxication.

Today is a typical summer day for most people in the world. I wonder what these fortunate souls are doing right now. I have a shot of relief just *thinking* about existence outside of my skin.

The relief dissipates.

Mom tells me it's time for my evaluation and leads me to a room with blue walls. I sit down at the table across from a brunette woman in her fifties who asks me if I want Mom to stay in the room.

"No."

Mom nods and smiles like she's dropping me off at preschool then closes the door behind her. The woman gives me a piece of paper and says to draw a vertical line across it.

"Now, what I'd like you to do is make dots for all of the major turning points in your life," she says.

I don't have enough life in my body to even speak. I draw a line and make the first dot for my parent's divorce. I make dots for Todd moving in with us, becoming a Christian, going to college and then graduate school, suffering a bad break-up, landing my job as a psychological counselor, and getting on Klonopin. I look at the timeline.

Oh yeah, I forgot about Mom getting remarried. I insert that on the line.

"Now," she says. I'd like you to think about the next dot, the one that hasn't happened yet. What do you think that turning point could be, one that would get you from where you are now to a place of hope?"

"I don't have any hope," I respond.

The exercise is clever, though.

"What would it take for you to have hope?"

"Sleep. The only thing I want is sleep." I say it listlessly. I'm as capable of generating hope as I am of dancing in the rain and waiting for the storm to pass.

She looks at me without speaking for what seems like a little while.

I think I've stumped her.

"The thing that keeps us looking ahead, toward that next turning point, is *hope*," she finally says.

"I won't have any hope unless I get some sleep," I say.

Yes, I've definitely stumped her. She is staring at me, and I know she's wondering what to say that could help me consider this "hope" thing.

"I encourage you to think of hope as something that can get you to where you're going next, whatever that next turning point may be."

197

"Okay. Thank you."

She leads me out to the front desk, and Mom takes me upstairs to the next stage of my evaluation. We sit near the desk of a perky and plump woman who begins firing questions at me about my psychological history.

The intake interview.

I've given many of these. Now I'm on the other side being asked the same questions I've asked others. I know exactly what questions are coming, and the answers to them don't matter.

I give incomplete responses about mental illness and addiction in my family. Mom is looking back and forth between me and her with expectant eyes. Now the woman is giving me a pep talk on how drugs can give us the ability to function and live a normal life.

"A few years ago I found a drug that worked for me, and now I can function with my mental illness," she says.

"Yeah, how *about* that?" Mom says to me, still looking like she won something.

The woman leads Mom and me back downstairs to a small and stuffy office to see the psychiatrist, our final stop and the one Mom is the most stoked about. He's a middle-aged man with whiskers.

Mom is holding her breath eagerly. It's the big moment, and she's determined to get what she came for. The woman hands him the results of my evaluation before saying goodbye. The psychiatrist is scanning the papers, but Mom interjects, too eager to wait for him to finish.

"Sir, we came all the way here to get Luvox. Her brother has Obsessive Compulsive Disorder, and she's having a lot of obsessive thoughts. She can't sleep because of this huge amount of Klonopin she was on. I just think that the Luvox will help her with the thoughts. It works for her brother."

He frowns and looks up from the paperwork.

"How long ago did you discontinue Klonopin?" he asks.

"I was on a five-month taper, then took the last capsule maybe a month ago," I say.

"Your insomnia is not related to the Klonopin then."

My blood is hot.

"Yes, it *is*. I have benzodiazepine withdrawal syndrome. It lasts an average of six to twelve months."

"There's no such thing," he says.

"Yes there *is!* The problem is, some doctors don't *know* about it!"

His eyebrows are scrunched down.

"If it's been more than a few days since you discontinued, then it can't be the Klonopin," he retorts.

199

"I have read lots of articles and even *books* on benzo withdrawal. You just don't *know* about it!"

I get up and race out of the office and then the building. I'm outside the door and surrounded by the wall of rocks, the desert terrain, and the highway that brought us here.

I *hate* that man. So much that I want him to take benzos and then suffer the worst withdrawal known to humankind. It's the *only* way he'd believe me. If he doesn't suffer from it, he won't believe.

He just won't.

The slim awning above the door blocks a smidgen of the oppressive heat. Mom is paying for the visit at the front desk that is visible through the glass door.

She comes out with her golden ticket, the Luvox prescription.

Back in the Yukon, I'm telling her how much I hate that doctor and what a jerk he is.

"Yeah, he really *was* a jerk. All I needed him to do was prescribe me that Luvox, though, and he did. So that's a good thing."

We arrive at the pharmacy—it's in one of the long shopping strips outside our neighborhood. It is cool and carpeted in here. Mom approaches the drop-off area with the Luvox prescription.

Suddenly I feel a slight wave of numb relief that I'm positive is related to the air conditioning.

The clock on the wall says it's 12:15 p.m. When I sat in a fetal position in the front room at 6:30 this morning, I didn't imagine I'd make it this far in the day. But here I am.

And that dreadful psychiatric visit is behind me.

"Mom, can we go to Subway on the way home?" I say. "I'm going to get a veggie sandwich with cheese. I'm done eating raw."

"Sure, if that's what want you want to do."

"I ate raw for weeks, and now I'm done. I need something familiar."

"Okay, sure, Honey. Let's do it."

"Thanks Mom."

We pull up to a Subway station near our sandscaped neighborhood.

"Mom, will you go in and order for me? I can't face anyone."

"Absolutely, Honey."

"I'll take a foot long veggie sandwich with all vegetables except jalapenos on honey oat bread. Also, I want triple

201

provolone cheese."

"Got it."

Triple cheese makes for one thick chunk.

A much, much needed distraction.

It's only 1:15.

"I'm *so* glad we got you that Luvox. I am positive this is gonna help ya."

"Mom, the only thing that will help me is sleep. There's no such thing as being in a good mood without sleep."

"The Luvox will stop that obsessive thinking."

"I don't have obsessive thinking. I'm just *awake* all the time."

"Why don't you take it now?"

"No! Not now."

"I'm gonna give you two at bedtime."

"Whatever."

"Wanna go to the flea market?"

"I guess."

The flea market is open every day in Clove Valley in a wide field in the blazing sun, and there's little relief from the heat except for an occasional drifting breeze.

Mom and I are back in the Yukon and arrive at the flea market's gravel parking lot.

Torment is literally pounding me.

The first row of tents has tables of homemade jewelry, essential oils, homespun clothing, and ceramic décor. Mom is into this set of ceramic frogs meant for sandscaped yards and patios. There's a baby frog, a medium momma frog, and a large papa frog.

"I just love these," Mom says to the woman in the tent. "How much are they?"

"You can get all three for ninety-five," she says.

"Oh, man, this is very tempting. Very tempting *indeed.*"

I'm baking and need to walk.

"Mom, I'm going to go over to the vegetables," I say.

"Wanna pick out some tomatoes for us?"

"Sure, I guess. How many?"

"Oh, I don't know... A couple big bags. Make sure they're nice and red."

I wipe my forehead sweat with the back of my hand and trudge toward the long row of farmers under their tents. The first tent is all tomatoes. The second is tomatoes and corn, and down the rows are corn, okra, peppers and more tomatoes.

This is the fourth tent of tomatoes, and so far they all look the same. Michael Jackson's *Beat It* is blaring from a stereo in a tent across the dirt path.

I danced in a ballet recital to this song when I was four, wearing a jean jacket, a blue and white striped Danskin, and white tights. When I was older, Mom told me she laughed hysterically when I moved out of sync with the other dancers.

The weight of despair is pounding mercilessly now. The song, the heat, the farmers at their stands, and the strange faces on the dirt path are the whole turning world, and I'm dizzy. Something is dawning, rising steadily within me, and floating atop this song. A girl in her early twenties is walking by the farmer's tents and sees my face. She frowns. Her legs are moving but her eyes are locked on mine. She's seeing something in my eyes, and I know what it is.

It's my realization that I'm not going to get better.

Showin' how funky and strong is your fight. It doesn't matter who's wrong or right. Just beat it...

My fate is falling on me like a giant steel ball. I was chosen for this end... for suicide. It's been written in the stars all this

204

time. But it waited until this moment to reveal itself.

Just beat it, beat it.
Just beat it, beat it.

It's a matter of how and when.

The girl's eyes are still locked on mine; my face is troubled. The magnitude of my realization doesn't prevent me from feeling humiliated by my expression.

I didn't suspect it. I now know that *no one* with this fate suspected it, until the moment it became clear—the moment I just had. They didn't suspect it when they played as children or hunted for Easter eggs or started school. They were just like me. And now... I am just like them.

The girl has walked past me now.

I can't get tomatoes after all. I make my way back to Mom.

"Audrey, hi. I got the frogs. I'm gonna go pull the Yukon up as close as I can to this tent, and this woman is gonna help me load them. Didya get some tomatoes?"

"No, sorry, Mom. I didn't get any. I don't feel well."

"Oh, okay. Well, I'll get 'em after we load the frogs in."

I follow Mom to the Yukon and deplore the idea of getting in it.

"Mom, I'm gonna wait here in the parking lot. Just swing

205

back through here when you have everything. I can't get in the Yukon. It's too hot."

"Okay, if that's what you wanna do. I'll be just about ten minutes."

I stand here in the dirt lot facing the farmers' tents nestled in the sand and contemplating my fate. It is up to me to figure out how and when I am going to die.

What I know for sure is that I will.

I was silent on the way home from the flea market.

Mom and I are back in our sandscaped yard and it's almost dark. The E.R and clinic visits replaced my morning walk, so I'm digging my bare feet into the sand by the gate to get a feel of nature while Mom reclines on a green lawn chair by the house.

Cool sand and caressing breezes lift me away from my sleepless mind and body, and I can almost feel detached from my condition in this moment as I have on other evenings. I thought when I got out of bed this morning that such moments of detached relief would never come again.

Mom is talking with Kelsey on the cordless. Now she's walking toward me.

"Audrey, Kelsey wants to talk to you."

"I don't think I can talk right now, Mom."

"Audrey, he really wants to talk."

"I don't want him to know how I'm doing."

"Well, he wants to know. And he really wants to hear it from *you*."

"I'll worry him, Mom. I can't do that to him."

"But he *wants* to know."

I take the phone.

"Hi, Augrit."

"Hi, Kelsey."

I want to declare my suffering, desperately. I want to get my thoughts outside of me, to someone that cares other than Mom. And I know he'll listen and pity me.

Yet I can't stand for him to know.

"Audrey, how are you doing?"

"I don't really want you to know, Kelsey."

"But I really want to know."

I want to say it out loud—I want him to help me share the burden of my fate.

"I haven't slept in weeks, Kelsey. I just want to die."

A few moments of silence on the line.

Suddenly, a sob bursts forth from his chest.

It hits me that the moments of silence on the line were him breathing in so that the sob would have room to travel up his chest.

My heart is cracking in two.

For the rest of my life, I'll never forget that sob. Now I wish more than anything that I hadn't said those words to him.

"I was moving the stuff you left here to the other side of the garage today, and everything just hit me all at once," he says.

I'm sobbing too, now.

"Kelsey, I don't want you to worry about me. I can't stand causing you pain."

"Don't think about me. It's just that... you've been dealing with this for a *long time,"* he says.

I had told Kelsey my situation back when I was searching for a drug to replace the Klonopin.

"I know, Kelsey, I know. I could still get better, though. Just takes time. I just got off the Klonopin a few weeks ago."

"Okay," he trembles. He doesn't sound hopeful.

"Audrey, I'll do whatever it takes! I'll get on a plane and fly there *tomorrow!*"

"No, it's okay, Kelsey. There's nothing you can do."

"I will! I will fly there!"

"It would just make me more miserable to be in this condition with you here."

"Okay... but... I *will* fly there if you need me to."

"No, it's okay, Kelsey. It wouldn't help. But thank you so much for thinking of me."

"I don't know what kind of terrible world this is we're living in!"

"I know... I don't either. I just don't want you to worry about me. I'll survive... I'll *try* to survive."

"But how long can a human being *go?*"

"Benzo withdrawal lasts an average of six months and then my sleep could come back."

I need him to think I have something that goes away over time.

"Okay," he whimpers.

We say we love each other, and I give the phone back to Mom. My heart is still cracking as I replay him breathing in and letting out a sob. Hurting him made me see how much I matter, how my staying alive is for him more than it is for me.

But it wasn't worth it.

It's ten minutes later and Mom comes back toward me with the cordless. This time, it's Della.

"Hi, Della," I say.

"Hi, Audrey, how are you doing?"

"Not good."

"Oh, I'm sorry, Audrey."

"Thanks, Della. How are you?"

I zone out some while she tells me about her life in Washington with her husband, T.J. That must not be what's really on her mind, though, because now she is crying. "Audrey, I'm just so sorry you're going *through* this."

"Thanks, Della. I just don't want you to worry about me."

"Oh, I won't worry."

She really won't. She doesn't worry like Kelsey does.

"Just pray for me, okay?"

"I will, Audrey."

When I give the phone back to Mom, she walks back to the green lawn chair.

The dogs are galloping around the yard but leaving me alone.

I close my eyes. The Michael Jackson refrain is echoing under the blinding sky across from the farmer's stands on the dirt path, and the girl is walking by looking at my face.

Showin' how funky and strong is your fight. It doesn't matter who's wrong or right.

I'd do anything to take back what I said to Kelsey, to rewind time and never hear that sob.

I was absolutely certain when the refrain played at the flea market that my fate was revealed—my life would end in suicide. Now Kelsey's silence, his sharp breathing in, and his heaving cry are piercing through the refrain. Here under the canopy of stars with my feet in the sand, my mind is muddled. I don't have any idea if I'm going to live or if I'm going to die. I don't know if I will even have a choice in the matter. I know one thing only, and that's that I love my brother more than I love me.

8 Maybe it was God

April 1990 LaPorte, Indiana

I gradually got over Buster. But not over death.

Apparently, my little brother was thinking the same thing.

Almost one year after Buster died, Mom asked five-year-old Kelsey to please put away his toys in the living room.

"Why? You just live and you die, and that's it!" he yelled. He ran out of the room.

That was the Saturday before Easter. Mom decided that Kelsey, Della, and I were living without hope. She reasoned that just because *she* didn't believe in God didn't mean we shouldn't.

"We're going to church tomorrow," she announced. "Todd, get the newspaper and help me pick one." He handed the worship section to Mom, and she found a listing for a church that met in a movie theater.

Still in pajamas on Easter morning, Della, Kelsey, and I grabbed our baskets and ran into the living room. Mom scanned the room with her video camera. We found plastic eggs with candy inside. I grabbed a large chocolate-covered marshmallow shaped like a bunny from the stone fireplace ledge and ate it for breakfast. I changed into a white dress with pink flowers and a straw hat. Mom had us talk to the camera outside, saying what we were looking forward to.

Mom was made up in red lipstick, mascara, and a navy dress with white dots.

Whew. One piece of clothing meant no clashing.

The breeze rustled the leaves on our biggest front yard tree as Todd beckoned us into the Suburban. It was a bright day on The Back Nine, like the one a year before when Todd led me down the hill to Buster's grave.

Entering the movie theater church was like going into a cave. I hated to leave the sunlight, but I liked the cool air inside. People hustled through the lobby in Sunday clothing, leaving trails of perfumes. Kelsey, Della and I were escorted into the theater for kids. The greeter pointed Mom and Todd to another theater, where there would be a sermon for adults.

We watched a puppet show with kids we didn't know. It was okay, though, not to know anyone, since the room was dark and the puppets were the ones lit up. The puppets enacted a story about women finding Jesus' tomb empty. They told some men it was empty, but the men didn't believe them.

I was dreaming about the Cadbury eggs I'd eat at Granddaddy's country club after church along with my aunts, uncles, and cousins. That place made me particularly happy.

Back at home that afternoon, Mom said she had an announcement. The only announcement she'd ever given us was that Todd was moving in. What would she announce now?

Mom told us to sit at the dining room table. She sat at the head of the table looking like a Kindergarten teacher ready to give us a lesson. Heavy earrings stretched the holes of her ears into long vertical lines. *Too* long. They looked like they might tear all the way through her flesh and drop to the ground.

I cringed.

"I have to tell you guys something. Something very, very important." she said, nodding. "Everyone listen very carefully."

I had a few butterflies.

But she didn't announce anything. "What did you learn at church today?" she said.

Della, a stutterer, said, "Jesus rose from the d-d-dead." Her pink and yellow puff-sleeved dress made the stringy tail still hanging down her back look out of place.

I remembered the puppet show. "Jesus rose from the grave. And when the women told the men about it, the men didn't believe them."

"Yes! That's right! Kelsey, what about you?"

"Jesus died for us," he mumbled, hunched over in a chair too large for his frame. Only his head, bowtie, and tips of his shoulders were visible.

Mom nodded and smiled. Todd stared at her wide-eyed across the table, wearing his Sunday outfit that matched Kelsey's: a white dress shirt and black slacks.

"Today," she said, "I heard some *very special* words in the sermon. I heard, "Jesus is the Son of God" and thought, *Why hasn't anyone ever told me this before?!* If Jesus really *is* the Son of God, and I now believe He is, my life has to *change!*"

None of us had anything to say.

"I need to get a hold of that *sermon tape!*" she erupted. "Then, I can listen to it, hear just *exactly* how that pastor put it, then explain to *everyone,* just the way he did, that Jesus is the Son of God. If only I can find out exactly what it was that pastor *said!*"

Still nothing to say. I was, I admit, a little excited. I wondered what would change. Would our lives at The Back Nine get better in some way?

215

The next Sunday, Mom purchased the sermon tape from a white tablecloth just inside the door of the theater. That night she tucked us into bed, reclined on her mattress, and listened to this tape she had waited seven days to get a hold of. She would find the words that changed her life, and then, she reasoned, she'd be able to change everyone else's.

The next night, Mom told us with dismay in her voice that the pastor, all the way through the sermon, never said the words she had heard on Easter Sunday: "Jesus is the Son of God."

She decided that part must have been edited out. After college, she worked at a radio station as a newscaster and knew very well the distinctive little snick that gave away an edit. She'd find that noise to prove the phrase had been taken out.

She listened to the sermon again. No noise. She listened to it for the third time. Still nothing.

"Todd!"

He appeared in the doorway like a butler. His legs stood like thin sticks under his baggy shorts printed with palm trees, a J.C. Penny clearance find of Mom's.

"Todd!" she said again, now that she had his full attention. "I listened to that sermon *three times,* and not *once* did that pastor say that Jesus is the Son of God! Not *once,* Todd! I

216

don't get it, Todd, I don't *get* it!"

Todd looked down to think. When he looked back up to meet her gaze, his eyes pierced the space just to her right.

"Maybe it wasn't the pastor that said it to you. Maybe it was *God*."

She looked at him and didn't blink.

Since the night Todd stood in the doorway, Mom has told us that God spoke to her in the movie theater Easter Sunday when she was 34 and said, "Jesus is the Son of God."

We had no reason to doubt her.

"Todd tried to tell me about Jesus," Mom would say. "But I hated Christians! I thought they were *freaks!* Now, I just wanna tell the *whole world* that Jesus is the Son of God!"

I imagined her trying to tell this to my aunts, uncles and cousins over lunch at Granddaddy's country club. I didn't see it going well.

PART III: THE WINNEBAGA

9 We're all gonna be in the winnebaga

July 2009 Clove Valley, CA

Mom has told us her stories so many times that, even though I was right there in them, I can't tell the difference between her stories and my memories. And the difference doesn't matter. It's all real, in our sinews, like the breeze bending the large trees on The Back Nine: Mom's belief that God has a plan for our lives.

I have lost my faith, but I cannot, *cannot* let my family lose theirs. Not on my behalf. If I harm myself, it will break their hearts and ruin their faith. I can't bear to ruin everything they've lived for up to this point, everything that keeps them going and gives them purpose.

When Mom and I came in from the sandscaped yard last night, she gave me two Luvox. Just as I didn't know whether I would live or die, I didn't know whether to take the Luvox. Did it even matter? I decided it didn't.

Mom was determined to watch me swallow it, and I didn't care to fight her.

My legs twitched all night long and were still twitching when I left the bed this morning. I went straight from my bed to the back yard to take advantage of the cool air while it lasted. A breeze trickled through the pine needles, and I fantasized I was in the Midwest and that my condition wasn't crippling, that maybe sleep wasn't necessary for a normal life. I dared myself to do some cartwheels in the sand. I ran and did a cartwheel, then another. *See,* I thought. *I just did two cartwheels. I'm fine.* Then I got dizzy, sat down at the glass patio table, and thought if I sat still long enough, my head would stop spinning.

But it didn't stop spinning for some time. I pondered the previous afternoon's realization that my fate was to die. Kelsey's sob replayed in my mind. I concluded I must die in a way that looks like an accident.

It absolutely *must* look like an accident. I cannot hurt my family.

It is late afternoon. I'm in the front room against the wall with my knees up and my hands around them—this position feels *quite* conducive for strategizing. My adrenaline is rising, and I feel the life rush back into me, to help me with my ultimate plan to end my life on this planet.

If only I was in nature, wild and free, far from this wasteland of manmade drugs; far from Mom, whom my presence is rapidly aging; and far from phones, so Kelsey would never have to hear my voice again. At night I could lie on the ground and hear the sounds of animals and rustling leaves and streaming water. Nature is a better *place* for people in withdrawal. I'd be alone with no one to bother, no one to blame, no one to hate.

Nature.

That's it! I could die of natural causes...

If Mom will drop me off in a wooded area, I can get lost and then die of hunger and thirst. By the time she picks me up, I'll have wandered far enough to be unable to find my way back.

The adrenaline is surging through me like a river, and I almost feel normal again.

I won't be culpable, because I won't be able to *find* food and water. I will look for them—my survival instinct will force me to. I will *try* to survive, but I won't be able to, and it won't be my fault.

"Mom, is there a wooded area somewhere around here where I could go hiking?" I call to the kitchen.

"Probably."

The afternoon is dragging, and I'm writhing in agony. I must execute this plan *soon*. If I can't get Mom to take me to a wooded area, then I will refuse food and water *here*—like a hunger strike.

Heck, I'll start now. If I know that death is where I'm headed, my adrenaline will stay up and I'll feel there's an end to this torment... And the adrenaline will help me persevere through the hunger and thirst.

The phone rings.

"Sweetie!" Mom says. Must be my stepdad on the line.

"Oh, really!" she says. "You found out! So where are we going? Quick! Tell me where we're going!"

His company must have told him where he's being transferred. Not that this affects me—I hope to not be alive four days from now. I think that's how long it takes to die from thirst. Hunger, I know, takes a heck of a lot longer, so the thirst will be the thing that does me in.

"Wisconsin? Oh, I am *so* happy! Alright, then! When do we go?"

Last time I had water was about two hours ago. I'm getting thirsty.

"Yeah, we're gonna *hafta* have the movers come the very day before we go and not a minute sooner."

My throat is dry. This is the time when I'd normally go get a glass of water.

"They'll hafta come for two days in a row then."

This thirst is getting pretty uncomfortable.

"All the animals will fit in the winnebaga. Oh, *man,* am I glad we bought that winnebaga!"

If a dry throat is *this* miserable, I can't begin to *imagine* a thirst so great it would kill me.

"Sweetie, just think, if we hadn't gotten that winnebaga, how the *heck* would we even get to Wisconsin with all the animals? There'd be no *way!*"

There is no chance I will endure this thirst. If sleeplessness is hell, dying of thirst on *top* of that is utterly unthinkable. I didn't think this plan through.

"We'll have just us, the animals, and our duffel bags. This is gonna be *fantastic.*"

My plan has a hole—a *big* one. I have tap water at my disposal just around the corner. Did I really think I was going to go through with this?

"Okay, Honey. Well, congratulations on the good news. I'll have a nice sandwich for you when ya get home. Love you."

Apparently, I'm not willing to do what it takes to die. I get up and walk into the kitchen for some tap water.

"Audrey, Honey, did you hear?"

"Yeah, I heard. Wisconsin. When?"

"About two months."

"Two months? Ha! There is no *way* I'll make it for two more months."

"*Yeah* you will. It'll be here before you know it."

If I am still alive in two months, I'll be shriveled up like a prune. Maybe Mom will have the pity to shoot me.

"So how are we going to get to Wisconsin?"

"In the winnebaga."

"How are the dogs and cats gonna get there?"

"They're going to ride with us."

She isn't serious. She can't be. But she does have two months to come up with a plan that's actually realistic... and humane.

"Five dogs and four cats, all in the winnebaga?"

"Yep."

"So, who's going to *drive* the winnebaga?"

"Your dad and I will take turns."

There she goes again calling him my dad.

"Wait... so what about me?"

"We're *all* gonna be in the winnebaga."

"You mean, all three of us *and* the animals?"

"Yep."

"How many days will it take to get there?"

"Oh, about five."

"Mom, the dogs and cats are going to slide all over the place... This is ridiculous! And how are they gonna use the restroom?"

"We're gonna stop and let the dogs widdle frequently, so no need to worry about that. Plus that living area and loft are just *so* nice. You wait n' see. It'll be *fantastic*."

"I won't be here anyway, so it doesn't matter."

"Yeah ya will."

"No I won't!"

"But you *will*."

"I won't if I don't wanna be!"

"These two month are gonna *fly*."

"If you think I'm gonna make it to Wisconsin, you're *crazy*. I'm not making it to Wisconsin."

"*Yeah* ya are."

226

She still thinks she can tell me what to do.

With each moment pressing me with unfathomable torture, two months is completely off the charts, wholly beyond measure. I will be long, *long* gone by the time they leave for Wisconsin. This California desert hellhole is my last stop, and there is certainly *no* existence on earth for me beyond it.

Going to Wisconsin in a winnebaga with my parents and their nine pets?

There is absolutely *no chance* that's going to happen.

Absolutely, positively, *none*.

Seven and a half weeks later

10 Strapped behind bungee cords

August 2009

The winnebaga looms high on the pavement of our driveway.

And there's my stepdad, standing outside it. He looks miniature in comparison.

The thing is *so* high, I keep glancing at it to make sure it really *is* that tall. Even the distant rock hills are blocked by its view. Not only are the wheels massive, but the floor must be thick and sturdy and the ceiling high enough to accommodate the loft. The sun in the sky is the only thing higher than the winnebaga, and that's only because it's eight a.m. By the time the sun lowers, we'll be long gone, probably not even in California anymore.

I can't fathom the thought of five days in that compact winnebaga with my parents and their pets. I won't have the morning walks to move my legs. I won't have the ability to get away from Mom or the animals.

Not to mention that Mom's backseat driving can't be rivaled—not even by a Hollywood movie.

I'm not entirely sure I'll make it through these next five days. Perhaps Mom will grant me lots of Subway stops and extra, *extra* cheese on my sandwiches for added distraction.

We are leaving "in an hour" according to Mom, and she put me to work sweeping the garage with this broom. I'm actually getting a break from the crashing waves of despair, first and foremost because the heat hasn't kicked in yet, and the winnebaga is giving ample shade to the sandscaped yard. Secondly, the repetitive sweeping motions on this cool cement floor are distracting, and I dare say they're quieting my mind a bit.

Moments like this, of almost relief, are all the more astounding each passing day. Minutes that didn't seem to move somehow became days, weeks, and now nearly two entire months. I really didn't imagine I'd still be here. In these last two months, my perpetually awake mind has traveled in more circles than I thought possible. Mom and I flew to Wisconsin and stayed for several nights in a hotel while she found a house. When we got back, I went with her to many stores as she picked out replacement tile and carpet for the house in Wisconsin she'd chosen. Those large stores were my opportunity to walk. I walked around and around the outside aisles while mentally justifying taking my life. After justifying it, I'd conclude I didn't really know if it was justified. I'd start justifying it all over again, and the cycle continued. Then there was the issue of how to accidentally die, and on that I made no headway whatsoever.

Day after day went by, and here I am. I won't miss California a single bit as long as I live. Wisconsin, not California, is where my life will conclude, and perhaps I will have the good fortune to catch a serious flu and die before winter.

Winter. My sensitive insides won't survive the cold. I'll have to wear a snowsuit just to step out and get in the Yukon.

The winnebaga has been in storage, and my stepdad got it out and parked it on our driveway last night. Mom was busy supervising the movers as they packed our house, wrapping each individual china plate and cup with layer after layer of paper, at Mom's insistence. Given how much moving she's done, I don't know why she'd want china-collecting for a hobby.

Last Saturday, my stepdad drove me to meet with the priest in La Joleta. I felt too weak to stand up long enough to be prayed for, and I almost canceled.

My stepdad said nothing as we crossed the railroad tracks right inside La Joleta, and I moaned about needing to die. It was a particularly oppressive day. There wasn't a cloud in the sky and everything looked like it was cooking. The Mustang windows were up and the air conditioning on, but the heat nevertheless seemed threateningly close, and I expected sweat to appear on my forehead. He waited in the parking lot as I went in for my two o'clock appointment for holy unction.

The priest beckoned me into his office, and I told him I was getting an average of half an hour of sleep per night.

"Oh, I can't imagine," he said.

I explained Klonopin withdrawal and the ineffectiveness of other drugs I had tried. "So prayer is really all I have to turn to," I said. "I am dependent on God healing me. So I figured I may as well get anointed with oil."

"I'm glad you did. Are you ready to ask the Lord to heal you?"

"Yes, thank you."

"Let's go and pray."

He led me through the foyer and into the nave up front by the icon of Christ. He dipped a brush in a small bottle of oil and swept the form of a cross on my forehead.

"This is blessed oil from the lamp which hangs over the relics of St. Panteleimon," he said.

"Oh, that's great."

I stood there as steady as possible as he prayed. He chanted Psalms then read the New Testament verses on healing and anointing with oil. He prayed from the service book, ending with this prayer:

"O Lord who, in thy mercies and bounties, healest the disorders of our souls and bodies, do Thou, the same Master, sanctify this Oil, that it may be effectual for those who shall be anointed therewith, unto healing, and unto relief from every passion, every malady of the flesh and of the spirit, and every ill; and that therein may be glorified Thy most Holy Name, of the Father, and of the Son, and of the Holy Spirit, now and ever, and to the ages of ages. Amen."

Then he asked the Lord to heal me from my insomnia, saying my name.

"Thank you," I said when he closed the book.

"I believe you will heal," he said. "I have *faith.*"

His tone revealed that he really did have it.

"I'm glad. Thank you for believing and for praying for me," I said.

"Audrey, will you give me a hand with something?"

I jolt. My stepdad has interrupted my thoughts. He is calling to me from just outside the winnebaga.

In my mind is the priest's face as I lean the broom against the side of the wall and take a giant step over the dirt pile I've created.

"I need ya to hold down some cords for me," my stepdad says, his hand around some elastic bungees.

I walk toward him, and he motions me to follow him into the winnebaga through its right side entry door.

We're both inside and eye-level with the bottom of the loft. On the table behind me is a hammer, skinny wall staples, and some more bungee cords.

"Okay, Audrey, this is what I need you to do. I'm going to nail the end of each cord, then I need you to stretch each cord across the loft. I'll nail the other side down, but I need you to hold it outstretched for me so it doesn't pull away when I'm nailing it."

"Okay."

"Got that?"

"I think so."

He's standing on the built-in "couch" and pounding the first staple over the bungee cord hook on the left side of the loft.

"Audrey, grab the end of this cord for me, will ya?"

"Okay."

"Don't pull it tight; just hold it out about right there."

I'm holding the cord close where his hand is gesturing.

"What are the cords for?"

"The cats are gonna be in the loft with the litter boxes, and we need to make sure it's real secure."

"So... the cats are going to be strapped in the loft behind bungee cords?"

"Yep."

"You have got to be kidding me."

"Nope."

"Whose idea was this?"

"Well, your Mom and I came up with it because we need a place that keeps the litter boxes from sliding and tipping over."

I'm not entirely sure they won't tip over up there. I hand him the second cord, and I hold the end while he nails the hook a foot above the first one.

At least the cats will be out of my way.

He nails three more cord hooks to the wood panel as I hold each end. He steps off the couch, grabs the first cord, and stretches it diagonally across the loft. He staples the hook in while I keep it stretched. He staples the next two cords below the first. He staples the last two cords across and above the other three. There are now five bungee cords stretched diagonally across the loft.

He steps back and studies the cords.

"Looks like we'll need at least two more, probably going straight across. I've got more bungees in that box in the garage if you'll go get 'em."

"Okay."

We're back in the winnebaga surveying the final design, and Mom comes in and joins us. She's dressed in khaki shorts and a sleeveless cotton shirt that shows the dry, orange-tanned skin hanging from her forearms. Her grey hair is in its usual messy loop on her head, and her sunglasses rest on her forehead.

Todd is in khaki shorts too, and his black t-shirt is tucked in and tight against his tummy, which sticks out just like it did when he used to be scrawny. Mom does a better job picking out his clothes now than she used to.

"Oh, wow! Good *job,* Todd!" Mom says. "We're gonna take off in 15 minutes, okay? Audrey, almost done sweeping the garage?"

"Yeah."

I head back to sweep the last of the dirt into the sand on the side of the house. I stroll into my bedroom and grab my black duffel packed with everything I brought here: Hanes clothing, toothbrush and toothpaste, a few rubber bands, my icons, and what's left of the beeswax candles from the thrift store.

I get to the winnebaga in time to see Mom handing Todd the litter boxes one by one. Todd is stretching aside an opening between two cords that's wide enough to push the litter boxes through. Now Mom is going inside to get the cats. She comes back out with Dinky in a small cage.

"Okay, Todd, now I'm not gonna open this cage until you are ready to *immediately* grab Dinky and push her between the cords... Okay, Todd, here's Dinky... *Quick!*" she says.

Todd grabs Dinky with his right hand while keeping two bungee cords stretched with his left. He lifts Dinky up and through the opening in the cords.

They repeat the procedure with Snowball, Pumpkin, and Cuddles. All the cats are now sprawled out on the loft.

Now for the dogs.

I'm going to be the last one in the winnebaga for three reasons. One, I don't want to be in it a second longer than necessary. Two, I need to get fresh air while it's still possible. Three, if I'm already in the motorhome when the dogs tumble inside, they'll stampede towards me slobbering.

Mom goes back in to get the dogs—they're all that's left inside. Last night Mom and Todd packed everything in the winnebaga that wasn't taken by the movers.

Mom opens the front door to the house and the dogs bound into the winnebaga—no coercion needed other than Todd's gesturing hand. There's nothing they like better than going for a ride.

Traveling across the country in a motorhome is the dogs'

idea of a good time, even if it isn't mine.

Before I get in behind the dogs, I notice the back of the motorhome.

"Mom... it's called a *Winnebago*... with an *"o."* Why do you guys call it the *'winnebaga?'"*

"Oh, I don't know, Honey, that's a good question."

"Yeah... it *is* a good question. So... what's the *answer?*"

"Well I don't know *what* the answer is. The winnebaga is just what we call it... Alright, *everyone in!*"

She closes the door behind me then climbs into the passenger seat.

June 1990 LaPorte, Indiana

That summer, Todd had "become friends with a troublemaker" and ended up at the Sherriff's department. Todd was allowed to make one call and said he wanted to call Mindy Malone.

"What's your connection to Miss Malone?" asked the Sheriff.

The Sheriff knew that Mom was Judge Malone's daughter. Judge Malone was well-known in the town—he had run for congress in the 60s. Todd reasoned that having a connection to Mindy might prompt the sheriff to let him go.

"She is the woman I am going to marry," declared Todd.

The sheriff dialed up Mom and told him he had a man named Todd Morgan with him.

"It's nothing serious," he said. "We're just asking him some questions about his acquaintance. Ms. Malone, Todd mentioned he is going to marry you. Is that true?"

"No, no, it's not. It's *certainly* not," she chuckled.

Mom picked up Todd and brought him back home.

Mom couldn't picture herself with a wiry, cross-eyed guy from the poor side of town, thirteen years younger, without money or education. But she didn't have plans for him to leave. She liked the way he played with us.

"He is *so* good with you kids. Isn't he *so* funny?" she said when he played the tickle monster with us.

The second-most thing she liked was his attention.

On an afternoon later that summer, Todd kissed Mom when she was leaning against the wall as I walked toward my bedroom. My walk became a dash.

They probably saw me, but I pretended I hadn't seen anything. I wondered how long it would be before Mom married one of the lawyers or doctors Granddaddy was always encouraging her to go out with. Todd would be

241

crushed. Not only that, but he probably wouldn't be able to live with us anymore.

I bet Todd would be really sad if he had to stop living with us.

Mom had bought a tape of an 'a Capella' band from a lady sitting at the white cloth table at the movie theatre church.

"An a Capella band is a band that doesn't use any instruments. Just their voices," explained Mom.

"You can't even tell they aren't using instruments!" I said.

We listened to the songs again and again whenever we were in the Suburban. Soon, we could belt out the lyrics together. We sang them on the way to church, then we sang them again on the way from church to the supermarket deli.

"Roll the stone away, roll the stone away. Lord God Almighty's gonna roll the stone away. He promised He'd rise up on the third day! Lord God Almighty's gonna roll that stone away."

I felt a rush when we sang, like adrenaline along with happy memories of snowmobiling, eating pizza and going to Granddaddy's country club. Maybe this Lord God Almighty had power, even more power than the things that didn't feel good, like Buster's lifeless body.

September 1990 LaPorte, Indiana

Todd was invited along to family gatherings at Granddaddy's and at my aunt and uncle's house.

Granddaddy gave Todd ever more projects do to around The Back Nine. Todd got the snowmobile going in the winters. In the warmer months he landscaped and broke up fights between the stray dogs we accumulated after Buster died.

Todd had lived with us three years when Mom made another announcement while we were all at the dining room table in early fall.

"Todd and I have decided to get married," she said. "God doesn't care about age. God cares about the heart."

My face flushed. That summer day—the day Todd kissed Mom—was the biggest piece of evidence they were more than friends. I'd pushed it out of my mind, pretending it hadn't happened. Now at last the secret was acknowledged in the open.

Well, at least the awkward announcement was over with.

Todd *might as well* marry Mom—that meant he was never leaving. It didn't appear he'd be leaving anyway, and by that point, I didn't want him to leave. What would become of us if he left?

243

Della and Kelsey belted out "yays" and "horrays."

I followed their yells with, "That's great," and I really meant it.

Mom told Granddaddy the news on the phone that night. He told her to come over to his house in the morning.

On the way to Granddaddy's house, past working class neighborhoods and the supermarket where Todd worked, the scenery became brick homes with ivy crawling up the sides. Granddaddy's house was across the street from a parochial school with an iron gate. Mom was raised in that house from birth.

Granddaddy collected Asian art, his favorite, during his overseas travels with the family when Mom was a kid. In his living room above the fireplace was a mural of an Asian man, plump like the Buddha, leaving a trail of flower petals. Another Asian man was printed on the folds of an ivory fan that sat on the wooden side table.

Mom told us to play downstairs while she talked with Granddaddy. We headed that way, but I stopped on the top step.

Granddaddy sat down and hunched forward on the antique chair next to the fan. Mom sat on the couch across from him.

Judge that he was, he stroked his chin in intimidating silence before his opening statement.

"What are you doing with this *young stud?*"

It didn't sound like a question.

Todd wasn't a stud, and we all knew it. But this wasn't the time to remind Granddaddy.

"I cannot *begin to imagine* what I'm going to tell my friends when they see my daughter with this *young stud,*" he continued. "He's got no money, no education, no future. This is going to *kill* me."

Mom understood.

"I want you to end your relationship with Todd," the judge concluded.

Mom repeated the news. "Todd and I have decided to get married. He loves the kids, he loves me, he loves The Back Nine. And I love Todd. He is just what we need. God brought him to us."

My grandpa twisted his face like it could wring the stupidity from her words.

"My *god,* Mindy. You say this has to do with God? My *god,* let's look at the facts. Todd doesn't have an education. He doesn't have money. He's practically a kid. *Dammit,* Mindy, you are throwing your life away."

Her lips tightened but her voice didn't change.

"I am happy, Todd is happy, the kids are happy, and that is all that matters."

His face twisted some more.

"This will *ruin* me. What am I going to tell my friends? What am I going to tell my friends when they ask why my daughter is with this *hired hand?*"

"Daddy, I don't expect you to understand. You gotta accept it, but you don't have to understand it."

The judge shook his head with refusal.

"If you marry him, I will *die.*"

November 1990 LaPorte, Indiana

Granddaddy arrived at The Back Nine and waited for Todd to get off the golf cart. It was late fall, and the sun was bright but the air was cool. Della, Kelsey and I were playing in the park across the driveway. We started making our way over to say hello. Todd hopped off the cart as Granddaddy approached him.

"I need to have a word with you." He motioned Todd into the barn.

They went in through the side door nearest to our little gray house. The barn had three large sections, each with its own sliding metal door. The middle section housed Granddaddy's old and dank R.V. that smelled on the inside like it had never been cleaned. The other sections held tools, mowers, old gloves and supplies.

It looked like Todd was about to get in trouble with Granddaddy. The middle sliding door was cracked open and let in a long path of sunlight that brightened the spot where they stood.

Granddaddy's head was bald other than tufts of white hair above his ears. He stood wide like a toddler to keep his old frame balanced. He pulled a check from the inside pocket of his blazer and held it in front of him. Dust swam in circles in the sunlight above the thin strip of paper.

"Listen, Todd. I am holding in my hand a check for ten thousand dollars."

"K." Todd's eyes gazed off-center, but that didn't detract from his focus.

"I am going to give you this. This will be a good start for you. But there is *one* condition."

"What's that," said Todd.

"You need to leave town tonight. You need to leave LaPorte and not come back. You cannot see Mindy again. You cannot come back here under *any* circumstances."

Todd looked down.

"Uh, I can't do that, sir."

"The *hell* you can't! I hired you to take care of this property. I pay you a good sum. I have never been unfair to you. I am asking you to do this for me and for the sake of my grandkids. *Leave town.*"

"I can't take that money. Mindy and I are going to get married. I realize you don't like it, sir."

Granddaddy's eyes glared. His lips curled under in a scowl. He stomped back to his Volvo shaking his head like he could make the world spin away from him.

Todd and Mom made wedding plans in secret. They would be married the Saturday after Thanksgiving, when Granddaddy would be with family on the east coast. The man who gave me piano lessons was married to a woman pastor of a Pentecostal church, and Mom gave her a call. Her name was Shirley.

Mom and Todd met Shirley in a musty sanctuary a couple miles from home.

"Before I can agree to marry you," she said, "I need to know if you have the Holy Spirit. Let me ask you something. Do you speak in tongues?"

"I do," said Todd. He looked at Mom.

"Well, no, I don't," she said.

Shirley was large and strong with bleached blond hair. She leaned forward and gripped her thighs with meaty hands and said, "We need to ask the Holy Spirit right now for the gift of tongues."

248

Tongues didn't come after fifteen minutes of Shirley's pleading, so she ordered Mom to try at home. Todd had borrowed a book of Goldy's about the gift of tongues. Mom read it and learned how to pray for the gift. She opened her mouth and spoke gibberish, as the book recommended. It had promised the Holy Spirit would take over from there. But He didn't.

"I have my reservations about this marriage," Shirley said at their second meeting. "A good foundation for a marriage requires that both of you be *true* Christians."

Mom said, "But I must have the Holy Spirit. God spoke to me in that movie theater. How could He speak to me if I didn't have the Holy Spirit?"

Shirley must have thought that was a good point. At the end of the meeting, she agreed to marry them. She reasoned that since Todd spoke in tongues, this might help sanctify Mom.

A lover of Danskins, Mom bought matching long-sleeved black leotards for herself, Della and me. She found purple fabric with a tropical flower print. She got to work on her sewing machine to prepare for the wedding day, making matching skirts for the three of us. With the same fabric she made a tie and bow-tie for Todd and Kelsey along with handkerchiefs to hang from the pockets of their suit jackets.

The cloudless, autumn morning after Thanksgiving of 1990 was bright like other important days on The Back Nine: the day Buster was buried, the day Mom told us she heard the voice of God in a movie theater, and the day Todd didn't take the check from Granddaddy in the barn.

We posed in matching outfits in front of our paisley green couch so that Missy, Mom's best friend since childhood and one of the five wedding guests, could take a picture.

"I am *not* marrying you in navy blue socks!" Mom said to Todd after the photo.

Todd changed into black socks to match his suit and shoes.

The sanctuary was largely empty. The only guests were Missy, a couple who worked with Mom, Todd's best man who was a member of his Bible study group, and Granddaddy's housekeeper Gina. Gina knew better than to tell Granddaddy about the wedding before he got back from his vacation.

My face swelled red as I stifled a laugh while walking down the aisle in my leotard and fuchsia flowered-print skirt. A song by Twila Paris blared.

How beautiful the hands that served
The wine and the bread and the sons of the earth
How beautiful the feet that walked
The long dusty road and the hill to the cross
How beautiful,
How beautiful,
How beautiful
Is the body of Christ.

After the wedding, we and the guests went to our house for fried chicken.

Granddaddy returned from his Thanksgiving vacation the next day. True to his word, he got into his bed "to die" after Gina told him Todd had married Mom.

When Mom didn't hear from Granddaddy the week following the wedding, she called his house.

Gina picked up.

"No, you cannot talk to him! He is *dying,* and it's your fault!" Her thick Spanish accent housed an accusatory tone.

"*Please* let me talk to him."

"You cannot talk to him! He has laid down to *die!*"

Granddaddy lay in bed for another week before he got up and back into his routine. Pretending a wedding hadn't happened, he was again on The Back Nine with more projects for Todd.

Not much changed—Todd had been living with us for three years before the wedding day. He'd become a part of our family long before he married Mom.

He coached Kelsey's basketball and little league teams. He drove me through neighborhoods as I sold Girl Scout cookies door-to-door. He packed our lunches, took us for hayrides around The Back Nine in the fall, and took us to doctor's appointments.

251

My friends' fathers and stepfathers were not mistaken for teenagers, as Todd was. But Todd was the father I had. He made life at The Back Nine fun and adventurous. Over time, I forgot he had once been a stranger. He was the man in my life. He held Mom together. And that held us all together.

Eventually, I said, "G'night, Todd. Love you," and hugged him goodnight, avoiding eye contact while heading for the stairs.

"I love you, too, Sweetie."

I saw him cry a couple more times: first when his dad died and, two years after the wedding, when Goldy died.

Mom went to Goldy's house for the very first time after her funeral. We needed to help Todd go through her stuff. Mom saw firsthand that this woman she'd refused to visit had lived in poverty and pain.

Mom saw the metal spring popping up through the cushion of the couch. She saw the quarter still jammed in there.

"Oh, my gosh! Goldy put that quarter there so the spring wouldn't poke her back!" said Mom.

She took just one of Goldy's belongings for herself... the cardboard with hunter green fabric and fuchsia embroidered lettering that said, "God Answers Prayer."

That night, Mom asked Todd to tell her more about Goldy. She learned that Goldy prayed every day as Todd was growing up that he would someday have a Christian wife.

Mom was dumbfounded, like the night she listened to the sermon tape and never heard the words "Jesus is the Son of God."

She told us kids the next day.

"Todd wanted to marry me, so God made me a Christian! He did it for Goldy!" she said.

"So you think you are a Christian because Goldy prayed for you?" I asked.

"There's no doubt! It's the only explanation!"

"Just think," I said. "A woman who lived in the poorest section of town, with a grandson you could have babysat for, is the reason you're a Christian. And you are the reason me, Della, and Kelsey are Christians. It's all because of Goldy."

"*Yes! Yes!*"

August 2009 Outside Clove Valley, California

"Todd, I'm telling you. We go North on 75 for just two more miles before the Interstate."

"Mindy, the Interstate is 45 miles east. You are thinking of Highway 9. But we are not going to take that. It doesn't get to Route 74."

"No, Todd, *no!* Get over to the right!" Mom is shrieking and pointing toward the upcoming exit.

"Mindy, you gotta *stop*. I looked at the map on the Garmin this morning. I *know* where we're going." His lips are tightened into thin lines.

Mom's eyeballs scan the side and front windows of the winnebaga in such rapid cycles that they're mimicking an oncoming seizure. Her hands are thrashing. "Oh, no, Todd. Oh, *no!* Listen, you need to trust me on this one. You need to get over to the right *right now!* Take the Interstate, and then we will pull over and look at the Garmin together. Quick! Put your turn signal on! You've gotta get in front of that Ford Explorer!"

Todd doesn't say another word, but he's shaking his head back and forth and chuckling dryly. He looks into the right rear-view mirror then veers up and to the right until he's in front of the Explorer.

I am slightly elevated, sitting at the edge of the RV's tiny living area, and below are Mom and Todd in the driver and passenger seats. My head is just above theirs, so Todd's frustration and Mom's hysteria are directly in my vantage point. My left hand is gripping Todd's head rest and my right hand is gripping Mom's. I dare not touch Mom's arm, given her stress, but I need to grab onto something to ground me in my moment-by-moment decision to stay alive. My whimpering is low enough to minimize its intrusiveness but detectable enough to send the message that I need their attention.

Todd puts his turn signal on for the second time. There are two more lanes he still needs to cross if he's going to make it onto the exit.

"Todd, *Todd!* Don't *go* yet! You don't have room to get over the next two lanes! You're not looking in the mirror! Don't you see that van?"

"Mindy. I'm gonna tell you this just *once*. I can see *just fine*. You gotta *calm down.*"

The left corner of my eyeball glimpses the entourage in the living area behind me. Fuzzy is apprehensive but trying to lie still on the driver's-side couch. Tiny is lying on the floor, and Peanut is resting against Tiny's stomach. Zoom Zoom, large and lanky, is skidding as he paces up and down the aisle between the table and couch. Misty is sitting tight against the bathroom door.

I lean my head back, and up above are the four cats, unmoved by the chaos. They're resting on the comforters in the loft, content with their view through the side windows and the security of two litter boxes. They are indeed barred from falling off the loft by the web of bungee cords stretching in all directions.

I admire Todd's ingenuity.

I'm also one hundred percent certain this is the first time in history cats have been strapped behind bungee cords in a winnebaga loft.

Not ninety-nine percent.

255

One hundred.

Todd is successfully onto the exit Mom demanded he take. We pull over at the first gas station to the right off the highway. Todd examines the map on the Garmin to verify the best way to route 74. Mom now trusts Todd to find the answer because she has scooted next to him to verify he's finding it. Her lips are no longer jutting forward and her eyeballs have stilled. Her diaphragm is rising and falling slowly as her breathing has returned to normal.

"We better let the dogs widdle," she finally says.

This is about the worst news I could hear.

"Mom! We have only been gone for twenty minutes! Are we going to stop and let them use the bathroom *every twenty minutes all the way there?!*"

We will never, ever get to Wisconsin at this rate... which serves to support my original premise that I'm not going to make it to Wisconsin.

"No, Audrey, no. They can go a few hours. But they just ate before we left. Come on, Zoom Zoom. Let's go!"

"Mindy..." Todd protests.

"Todd, put the Garmin down and help me. We gotta take them out one at a time. You get in the back and restrain the others while I get Zoom Zoom on the leash."

"Oh, my gosh..." I put my head down. Tears accumulate and

fall down my cheeks.

Mom leaves the passenger seat and makes the giant step up into the living area while I move out of her way. Todd exits from the driver's seat door and walks around to the side door. He opens it.

"Todd! You can't just *do* that! They are all at the door ready to run out! You've gotta be more *careful!*" Mom says.

"Mindy, I *got* it! They're not *going* anywhere."

Todd is pulling the door against his side so that the slim opening allows only him to squeeze through. He shuts it behind him. Mom moves over to the door and holds her body against it even though it's latched. Todd motions Tiny, Fuzzy, Misty and Peanut toward the back while Mom puts Zoom Zoom on a leash. Zoom Zoom's ears perk straight up and his eyes roll back. "Come on, Zoom Zoom," Mom goads. "That a boy. There ya go. Mama's gonna take you potty."

The word "potty" compounds my misery. I put my head in my hands. Even if I *could* sleep, I'd still want to jump off a bridge. I'll be hearing the word "potty" many times over these several days, and I won't be able to run away.

Mom is tumbling out of the winnebaga behind Zoom Zoom, and Todd's putting leashes on Peanut, Tiny, Misty and Fuzzy to get them ready for their turns.

It's been about two minutes, and Mom's pushing Zoom Zoom back up the metal stairs into the motorhome. Todd says to her, "I'll take Fuzzy and Tiny at the same time. You take Peanut." He's handing Peanut to Mom. Peanut's leash is hanging from his collar and dragging on the ground. Mom has her arms stretched out, and below her sunglasses her mouth is as close as it gets to smiling when she's stressed.

"Oh, *Peanut*. What a *handsome boy* you are. Come to Mama!"

Todd shuts the door behind Mom and is grabbing Tiny and Fuzzy by their leashes. "Audrey, go ahead and open the door for me when I tell you to... Okay... *Now!*"

I open the door. Todd is yanked, first by his left arm, then by his right, as Fuzzy and Tiny scramble down the metal steps and onto the dead yellow grass that borders a gas station.

Out the window is a view of the overgrown grassy knoll interrupted by the chaos of Mom and Todd and the dogs. Misty is still back by the bathroom awaiting her turn. Fuzzy and Tiny are leaping inharmoniously, jerking Todd's arms and legs in awkward directions. Peanut and Mom are ten yards to their right.

"Peanut, *widdle!* It's time to *widdle!*" Mom urges the Chihuahua. The passenger window is cracked just enough for some sound and a little hot air to stream in but not enough that a dog or cat could squeeze through—Mom's rule.

I wonder if the gas station worker is getting a view of this.

"Good *boy*, Peanut!" Mom says. She picks him up and kisses him on the snout then comes back in through the side door carrying him.

"Audrey, here, take Peanut. Set him down real gentle. *Gentle*, now. I'm gonna grab Misty and take her potty and then we can go. You wanna run in and getta snack?"

"No thanks."

Staying in here allows me to fantasize that this stop never happened to begin with.

Mom takes Misty back out onto the grass and passes Todd, who's almost back. He opens the door and keeps hold of the leashes while Tiny and Fuzzy tumble in, bringing with them waves of warm California air.

This misery is too great to be quantified, but I nevertheless have preferences. I prefer cold to hot air; I prefer no pets; and I prefer a vehicle that's moving to a vehicle that's stopped. As long as we're moving, I have that illusion that I'm traveling to something ahead on the horizon.

Something involving permanently exiting this winnebaga.

Just as I dreaded, the wave of despair is hitting even harder now that I don't have the option of trudging to a park and pacing around a grassy perimeter. I'm keeping my grip on Mom and Todd's head rests while looking toward the sky.

A view through the front window is imperative—I must, *must* at least *see* nature since I can't be in it. The sky ahead looks to be a destination point the winnebaga is reaching for,

259

which gives me the sense I'm leaving the present behind me. I want to shed each moment in this motorhome as if it is a layer of snake skin. But, again and again, I cannot.

My agitation is through the roof.

I whimper a little louder. I need Mom and Todd to care, to join me in my heroic feat of staying alive.

Mom's lips tighten inward ever so slightly.

Oh, no. Her compassion must be wearing thin, not least of all because she's continually worried about the dogs and, more specifically, the state of their bladders. She's not thrilled that my plan as a passenger is to sit directly behind her and Todd and whimper.

"Mom, I'm not trying to be obnoxious. I just really need you two to have compassion. This is really, *really* hard for me. I don't know how I'm gonna make it through this trip."

"Why not just have a seat on the nice couch back there," she suggests.

She used the word "nice" rather than "fantastic," which means she's not in a great mood.

"No, I'm not sitting anywhere back there. The dogs are gonna climb on me and slobber!"

"*Okay* then."

I lower my whimpers.

The sun blazed without a cloud all morning. Now it is mid-afternoon, and light clouds have joined together and stretched over the whole sky. Perhaps clouds are one of the perks of leaving Clove Valley.

Lightning flashes. Thunder cracks like a whip and is rumbling. The gray horizon is rapidly becoming dark blue.

Not a whole second has passed since the thunder whip, and Fuzzy is almost *entirely* on my lap, using the force of his body to push my arms out of the way.

I tighten them to keep him from sitting on top of me, but he's strong and unrelenting.

"Fuzzy, *no!* Go away! Oh, my gosh!"

"Oh, Fuzzy is *terrified* of storms," says Mom. "He just wants you to comfort him."

"I can't have a hundred-pound dog on my lap!"

Fuzzy has succeeded in breaking through the barrier of my arms, and his torso and full weight of his body are resting on my lap.

"Oh, my gosh. Oh, my gosh," I moan. "I can't get him off me. He's too heavy. I can't do this!"

"Audrey, you're gonna *hafta* just go sit on the couch where there's room for him to be right next to you, and then you can pet him."

261

"Oh, no. I don't wanna be on that couch."

But I've got to get this dog off me. I writhe free and stand up, taking the one step required to get on the built-in cushioned couch. Fuzzy is so close behind me he may as well be surgically attached. On the couch, he puts his torso back on my lap. My legs, at least, are free and dangling on the ground.

"Oh, my word."

Fuzzy is whining quietly, scared as a little baby puppy, although he is the largest of all the dogs and, by the looks of his gray whiskers, probably the oldest. He's pushing his weight on me as if his life depended on it.

I pet his head with my right hand. The other dogs, unaffected by the storm, are sprawled on the floor resting.

Lightning flashes and thunder cracks again across the dark sky.

"No *passing,* Todd! What do you think you're doing? Do you realize how *big* this thing is? You really think you're *not* gonna kill somebody going the speed you're going, with all this rain? What are you *thinking?!*"

"Mindy, I checked *both* mirrors before I put the turn signal on. Ya gotta *chill out,*" he says.

"Todd, you gotta remember this thing weighs eleven *thousand* pounds. Do not *pass* cars in the rain! Don't *do* it!"

"Mindy, I'm *fine.*"

"If you think you're *not* gonna kill someone with this thing, you're *dead* wrong."

The rain is lightening up.

"Audrey, we'll find a Subway after the rain stops, okay? Then the dogs can go potty without getting soaked. How does that sound?" Mom says.

"Good." That is, the part about getting Subway is good, but the part about the dogs going "potty" isn't.

"Are you gonna be okay for another 30 minutes or so? Then we'll stop?"

"Yeah."

Mom's been the one to go into Subway to order my sandwich, but she and Todd will be occupied taking the dogs out. And by "out" I mean another grassy knoll beside a public plaza. So I guess I'll be ordering my own sandwich.

"Okay, Todd, pull in here. Here, Todd, *here!* Where are you going? We can't pull in that close to the other cars!"

"Mindy."

"Audrey, wanna go in and order the sandwiches while the dogs widdle?"

"Sure, Mom, as long as you quit saying that word."

263

"Okay, while the dogs go *potty.*"

I put my hand over my face because I really might explode.

"No, Mom! *Stop!* I hate that word! Can you please stop using those words on this trip? I can't *deal* with this!"

"Todd, you want a veggie on wheat?" she says.

"That's fine."

"Okay, Todd and I want foot long veggies on wheat, no cheese."

"I thought you were eating all raw, Mom."

"Well, sometimes you gotta do what you gotta do."

"What happened to eating one *hundred* percent raw?"

"It's just too hard on this trip. But we're definitely staying away from the dairy cuz that's *critically* important."

"You guys want all the veggies? Even jalapenos?"

"Yeah, all of 'em."

"Vinegar and oil for the dressing?"

"Sounds good to me," Todd says.

Mom hands me a fifty dollar bill, and I walk into Subway.

I wonder if my mental state is detectable to the Subway patrons. I look normal enough, wearing the same thing I wore on my way to California—a navy Hanes t-shirt, gray Hanes drawstring shorts, flip flops, a low pony tail, and no makeup. But I'm being scourged and tortured within. Can I really stand here and order these sandwiches?

"What can I get you, Ma'am?"

"I'd like three foot-long veggie sandwiches; two on wheat, one on honey oat," I say.

That was the most civil interaction I've had since I was in Barbara's office watching the debris of my colon float down the tube.

"No cheese on two of them, double extra cheese on the third one."

I'm in the winnebaga tearing the paper wrap off my sandwich, and Mom and Todd are almost back in with the dogs.

Good. Let's get this show back on the road before the five-dog circus on the grass attracts too much attention.

The winnebaga is moving again, and I'm in my preferred position behind Mom and Todd. Fuzzy is asleep on the floor, the storm behind us. I chew each bite thoroughly because the crisp, flavorful veggies, sweet oat bread, and salty thickness of three layers of provolone make this sandwich the closest I'll come to pleasure within the confines of this motorhome.

265

The horizon is pretty as could be. The sun is out though the sky is still dark blue with storm clouds. Rays of sunlight shine diagonally and reflect on the wet highway. The beauty lends some relief and whispers that somewhere, up ahead, is a future that just may take me out of this torment.

Some way.

Somehow.

"Mom, are you still sure I'm going to get better?"

"Positive."

"Todd, what about you? Do you still believe my sleep will come back?"

"Yes, I do."

"How long do you think it will take?"

Todd shakes his head. "Hard to say, Augrit, hard to say. Just take one day at a time."

"Mom, do you think it will be a really long time till I heal?"

"No, I don't think it will be a really long time."

I won't probe further. If she tells me I'm going to heal soon, then I definitely won't believe her.

Dang it, this sandwich is all gone.

Mom picks up her cell phone and dials a number. "Yes," she says. "I'm calling to confirm our reservation for tonight. The name is Mindy Morgan... Okay, *fantastic*. Our estimated time of arrival is eight p.m."

Not that we want them looking out the window when we park an eleven thousand pound motorhome then let the dogs bound into their lot.

The sun is on its way down as we pull up in front of the Holiday Inn. I'm surprised this evening moved so efficiently. That feeling of the future being ever ahead stuck with me as I gazed through the front window. Mom spent the last hour reminiscing about her childhood, also a welcomed distraction.

Mom comes back to the winnebaga with the room keys. Todd drives us to the end of the parking lot and pulls into the space farthest from other vehicles.

This is the moment I've been dying for.

"Mom, I really, really need to take a *long* walk, for like an *hour*. Okay?"

"Okay."

"I'm just going to walk around the Holiday Inn. I'm not going to leave the parking lot."

Fresh, cool air. Setting sun. This is the only exercise I've had all day, and tomorrow it's back in the winnebaga.

I'm sauntering slowly back to the motorhome, and I believe it's been 45 minutes. But my energy is low, and I'm ready for the next thing, which is collapsing onto some clean white sheets, far away from any animals, and lying awake in the dark.

I enter through the side door of the winnebaga.

"Oh, Audrey, *careful!* Close the door behind you, *quick!* Come join us in here– it's like camping!" Mom says.

Mom and Todd are sitting in the living area, Mom on the couch and Todd at the table, with the dogs sprawled on the floor. Mom is holding a book about vitamins, and Todd is on his iPad checking work emails.

"No, thank you. I'm gonna go in the hotel room and lie down. Can you give me a key?"

"Oh, we'll come with you! We were just waiting for you."

"Who's 'we'?"

"You, me, and the dogs. Todd is gonna stay in here with the cats."

"The dogs are gonna be in the *hotel room* with us?"

"Yeah, I need to be able to take them potty at night."

Uh uh.

"This is crazy! All five dogs in the hotel room?!"

"That's right. Where did you think they were gonna sleep?"

"There is no *chance* I will sleep now! Not that I would anyway! But at least there would have been a *chance!* Now there's none, with all those dogs!"

"I'll keep them quiet, don't worry."

"Nooooooo!"

"It's the only option we have, Audrey."

"Does the Holiday Inn even *allow* pets?"

"This one is pet-friendly," she says.

"What's *that* supposed to mean? What's the pet limit?"

"Oh, probably two... I decided it was better not to ask."

"Mom, when they say they're pet-friendly, this is not what they have in *mind!*"

So much for a quiet room and a prayer for sleep. That prayer certainly won't get answered tonight.

Mom closes her book and stands up.

"Come on, boys! Let's go! Todd, can you help me get their

leashes on?"

"Mom, can I have the key now? I just wanna go in the room."

If I can beat them into the room by even *one minute,* that's one minute of quiet I won't have otherwise.

"Sure, here it is. Todd and I will be close behind you."

I'm on the full bed nearest to the bathroom, and Mom is on the bed by the door. Only she's hasn't spent much time *in* bed; I swear every fifteen minutes she takes another dog outside. Mom's whispers and the panting of dogs have been whirling around the room for hours.

"Misty, Misty, come on, girl, that's right. You all stay back. I'm coming right back," Mom says.

Mom's "whispers" are as crisp as an apple. She may as well use her regular voice.

The door squeaks, and there's a pitter-patter of paws all around the room. I open my eyes a crack, and no wonder— Zoom Zoom is galloping around the perimeter of the room in the excitement of Misty being outside.

"Misty, that a girl. Go potty. Go potty."

Mom is outside on the cement walkway, yet she's as audible as if she were beside me.

I'm stumped whether this night would be better if it slowed down or if it sped up. I desperately want this whispering and galloping to stop and just as desperately want to not set foot back in that motorhome.

It's getting close to sunrise; the sky out the window is a lighter navy. Not much time till Mom will tell me I need to get up.

She's actually still and quiet on her bed. Apparently, Mom stopped worrying about their bladders long enough to fall asleep. The dogs are still, too. They're lying on the floor sacked out.

Guess I'll close my eyes and see if something resembling rest is possible before Mom bounds out of bed.

Real moments of silence... Now I want time to hold still. I'm in no rush to get back in that winnebaga.

Fuzzy barks.

Oh no...

He barks again.

Oh please stop. Please, please, please. Why can't we have some uninterrupted silence?

"Woof! Woof, woof, woof!"

"Mom!"

But she already hears the barking. She lifts her head.

"Fuzzy, *cut it out!*" she says.

But he's *not* cutting it out. He's still barking.

Tiny starts howling.

I sit up in bed with my hands over my ears and watch.

Fuzzy's string of barks morphs into a wail. The other three join Tiny and Fuzzy.

I press my ears so hard they are starting to hurt.

The dogs are getting in a circle with their heads up. Their howls are rising to the volume of a siren every bit as loud as the one in the sandscaped yard in Clove Valley. Only they are five feet away from us in an enclosed space rather than in the open air. The volume is dangerously high—it may be doing real damage to my insides.

"Oh, my gosh, Mom, make it stop!" I say, but I know she can't hear me through the howls.

"Cut it out, guys, cut it *out! Stop* it! *Stop* it!" she yells.

They aren't listening—they're fully lost in their ritual. Not to mention there's no way they can hear her. An ambulance driving through the room would make less ruckus. There will be a knock at our door any second.

My heart's picking up speed. We'll get kicked outta here,

there's no doubt.

The blaring howls are reverberating and sending shock waves through my body. I am way too sensitive to bear this, and I don't have the stamina to gather my things and stumble out the door when the hotel manager kicks us out. And he *will* kick us out—the red digits on the bedside table say 5:17 a.m., and everyone in this building is undoubtedly wide awake from the noise.

My hands are on my ears tight as they can be, but that's not even muffling the sound. I hold my breath, hoping to still the inside of my body.

"No, *no!* Cut it *out!* Cut it out *now!*" Mom shouts.

I'm waiting for that knock.

"Mom, break them up!"

"No, Audrey, no! There's no *stopping* them! Boys, *boys!* Cut it out!"

One dog's enthusiasm is dying, and the others are following suit. Maybe they're getting tired.

"Stop it, boys! Stop it *right now!*"

The howls are slowing to pathetic wails, but I doubt the quieting down has anything to do with obedience to Mom.

Still no knock.

273

"Mom, they're gonna knock any minute. There is no way anyone in this hotel slept through that!"

"Boys, no *more* of that!"

The howling has died.

"Why hasn't anyone knocked yet? Mom, we're gonna get kicked out of here!"

"Well, we're leaving in an hour, so let's just hope we can make it here till then."

In an *hour?* So much for any significant stretch of peace and quiet.

The dogs are already lying back down, spent from exerting their energy and ready for a nap.

I have one hour, at most, of silence, and I hope against all hope for no interruptions. Unfortunately, this hour is going to fly by.

And it has. It's now 6:30, and at Mom's command I'm out of bed and dressed. I'm in a black and white Hanes outfit with flip flops. I may as well have been hit on the head with a bat, and I'm already fantasizing of exiting the winnebaga at the next Holiday Inn tonight.

The sunrise out the window is blinding.

"Audrey, wanna get some breakfast at the McDonald's down the road?" Mom says. "We can stop there on our way out."

"Yeah... Actually, can I walk there right now, and you guys can pick me up when you leave?"

"Sure, Honey." Mom hands me a ten dollar bill.

"Okay, thanks. I just really need to be outside and do some walking before I have to get in that horrible motorhome."

I open the door and step into the morning.

Ahhh, fresh air.

Even the sense I've been hit on the head is suspended as the yellow McDonald's arches loom tall, like a star that doesn't get closer as I walk toward it. My flip flops are treading on gravel while cars whiz by to the left. It's clear, and the morning air is cool.

The familiar combination of a city street and a morning sky is distracting, helping me almost feel normal as I trudge ahead, zoning out from my body and savoring this bit of nature.

I order two sausage biscuits and eat them before the winnebaga arrives in the parking lot.

11 A finite amount of colors

August 2009 Somewhere on the way to Wisconsin

What a hellacious day.

I'm holding onto Mom's shoulder. Every minute feels like ten—stopping no less than every two hours for the dogs to go out makes it seem we're not making headway. One gas station attendant gave us suspicious looks. When I went in to buy bottled water, she said we can't take our dogs to the bathroom on her property. I said I'd pass the message along to my parents. Problem is, the dogs were already "widdling."

It's only mid-afternoon, and there are several more hours to go till we stop at the next Holiday Inn.

"Mom, I can't stand this. I'm not going to make it to Wisconsin." I'm sitting in the same position as yesterday, my crossed legs at their headrests. My hand is gripping Mom's shoulder because I'm afraid my misery will spin out of control if I'm not touching her.

"Audrey, take a couple Luvox."

I yank my hand from her shoulder.

"No! Forget about that Luvox! It's *history!* I'm not going to take it!"

"Audrey, take some Luvox. It'll *help* ya."

It's been many weeks since I took one, but Mom has no intention of giving up and throwing out the bottle.

"I'm not putting that stuff in my body."

"Audrey, just please take two pills. I promise you'll feel better. *You'll* see."

"I'll take them tonight," I say.

But I won't.

"Take 'em right now then lie down on the couch. Maybe you'll even get a little nap in."

"A nap! Ha! You *know* I don't sleep!"

"I think you'll be surprised how much the Luvox helps."

"No! Leave me alone!"

We stop at a rest stop. Mom and Todd take the dogs out and I walk. Only a few minutes to exert my muscles and we're back in the winnebaga.

277

Todd has us on the highway again, and Mom comes back to the cabin of the winnebaga, opens up the cupboard, and gets the Luvox out.

She isn't going to stop until she shoves it down my throat. She hands me a new bottle of water and thrusts the pills at me.

"Audrey, here ya go. Now, take these."

She really is unrelenting, and I absolutely don't have what it would take to fight her.

I swallow two pills.

It's five p.m. and the winnebaga is steadily moving.

"What time are we going to be at the hotel?" I say.

"Seven."

"Oh, wow, seven? Then I just have to try and make it for two more hours."

When we get there, I'll take a walk, a long one, and then a warm bath that, if nothing else, will give me a break from the dogs. Then I'll lie down and hope against all reason for some semblance of quiet.

We arrived at the Holiday Inn at seven as Mom predicted.

It's 8:15; I walked around the hotel's perimeter then got the key from Mom, who is hanging out with the cats and dogs and Todd in the motorhome. The swipe card opens the door, and I set down my duffel bag.

I'm very dizzy now.

I don't think this is a normal kind of dizzy.

My thoughts are not making sense. They're jumbling, changing course. Yet I'm rational enough to stand back and notice.

Something's *really* wrong with me. Now I realize what—it's the Luvox. I didn't eat much today except one foot long veggie sandwich from Subway. Two Luvox was too much.

The bathroom. I need to get to the bathroom.

Here I am. This cool ceramic toilet will ground me. I sit on it—it's nice and cold even through my cotton shorts. This bathroom has light peach walls and a white floor tile. I'm gazing up into the crevices of the blotchy white ceiling paint.

The colors... the colors. There are only so many. A finite amount of colors... then they end. There's no more; they're finite. There's a lot, but then they run out. It's inevitable; they come to an end.

The colors spread out like a fan on the ceiling that meets the top of the peach wall. They are translucent, but nevertheless visible like a rainbow. The edge of the rainbow is the end.

279

I'm going to die. Just like the colors, I'm going to end.

You will take your own life... You will end, like the colors.

My cell phone is beeping from the side pocket of my duffel bag.

I tumble out of the bathroom. Other than the lamp on the table, the room is dim, and my duffel bag is on the floor next to the table.

My thoughts seem to be clearing. My phone says Marcia called. She and her husband Danny have called every few weeks since I left Kentucky. Other than Father Justin, Marcia is the only one I've picked up the phone for. I told her what had happened to me and that I thought the Klonopin did it. She believed me.

I have a voicemail from her.

"Hi Audrey, this is Marcia and Danny. We were just driving home from church and thinking of you. We just want you to know we are praying for you. Haven't heard from you in a while. We hope you will let us know how are you are doing. We love you."

The dizziness has gone. My thoughts make sense again. The colors in the bathroom—what was that? I had a delusion, I guess. What was that voice? It was telling me I had to die, to take my own life, and that I had no choice.

I dial up Mom on my cell.

"Mom, can you come here to the room?"

"Sure. Are you okay?"

"Not really. I had a weird experience. It was the Luvox. It's hard to explain."

"Okay, I'll be right there."

Mom opens the door, gets on the bed, and puts her arm around me.

"I was in the bathroom... something about colors. Colors run out... there are only so many. That it's inevitable I will take my life. It was a voice telling me I had to die. Then I got a voicemail from Marcia and Danny saying they were praying for me, right when I was in the bathroom. That wasn't a coincidence, was it?"

"No, *not* a coincidence," she says, looking in my eyes.

"I think the voice was the devil."

"Yes, yes."

"I think maybe God has a plan for me after all. Otherwise, why would Marcia call me right at that moment? Do you think God has a plan for me?"

"Yes, I absolutely do."

"That can't be a coincidence that she called me and was praying for me right when I heard that voice."

"No, it can't be."

"So you think God is watching out for me?"

"Yes, yes He is. He's showing you that."

"Yeah, I mean, I got the call from Danny and Marcia right when I heard that voice."

"Wow."

"Mom, you think I am going to heal?"

"Yes, I know you will. No doubt."

"Okay, Mom. Thanks for being there."

"You are so welcome, Honey. I love to be there for you."

"Mom, I'm gonna take a bath so I can get away from the dogs for a little while. That way, when they come in I will be already clean and in the bed."

"Sounds like a plan! You enjoy your bath. I'm gonna read in the motorhome with Todd for probably another 20 minutes, then I will hardly be able to stay awake. And then I'll bring the dogs on in."

"Okay. Thanks, Mom."

This water is quite warm, almost hot, and my wide awake body doesn't feel up for this submersion. I get out, dry off and put on a clean Hanes t-shirt, drawstring shorts, and white socks. Good thing I'm still in the bathroom because I hear Mom coming into the room with the dogs. There's Todd's voice, too. He's helping her bring them in.

If we're lucky tonight, there will be no howling.

I'm making a mad dash for the bed and getting under the covers. It's a little after nine, and I'm ready to lie down and savor the hours ahead that don't involve being in the winnebaga.

If the dogs will just stay out of my bed and keep the galloping to a minimum, a semi-peaceful night might be possible.

"I'm gonna go back out to the winnebaga and say goodnight to Todd," says Mom.

"Okay."

Fuzzy jumps up on my bed, and Zoom Zoom follows.

I sit up and push them off.

"Get down! No! You cannot come up here!"

They jump down, and it looks like they're staying on the ground for now.

Good. I am closing my eyes to shut the world out of my site, even if I can't shut my brain and hearing down. And there's plenty to hear: sniffling of snouts, pitter-pattering of paws on the carpet, and Mom coming back in then digging through her toiletries by the door.

Soon the lights will be off and the dogs may get drowsy. I sure as heck hope Mom doesn't take them out as often tonight as she did last night.

"Noooooooooo! Zoom Zoom, *nooooooo!"*

Her voice zaps my body. I clamp my hands over my ears and press them so hard that I don't know what's hurting my head more—her screams or my hands.

"Oh, no! Oh, no! No, no, *no!!!!"*

Whatever it is, I don't want to look.

But I *have* to look. Mom sounds like someone's been murdered.

I open my eyes and peer at Zoom Zoom in the center of the room. But he looks alive and well. Mom, though, is on the floor holding onto his body, and I don't get what the matter is.

"Oh, boy. Oh, boy. We've got a *real* problem here, Audrey! A *real* problem! You gotta *help* me!"

"Oh, no, Mom! Just tell me what it is!" My hands are still tight on my ears to muffle her voice.

"Zoom Zoom has eaten the Luvox! You gotta *help* me! Help me *right now!"*

"All of it? How do you even know he ate Luvox?"

I sit up in my bed and take my hands off my ears, and Mom's on her knees trying to pry open Zoom Zoom's mouth. Her elbows point outward, her face is in a childish grimace, and her grey hair is piled on her head in an especially tangled mass.

"Audrey, you gotta get down here! You gotta hold him so he can't move! I need to see if it's still in his mouth—Zoom Zoom, spit it out! Spit it *out!*"

I throw the covers aside, get on the ground on my knees behind Zoom Zoom, and hold his torso. Most of my weight is on his back. Mom's is squinting as she looks down his throat, her face severely contorted. She's holding his front and bottom jaws apart.

"Is there Luvox in his mouth?" I say.

"No. *No!* It's not there! He's swallowed it. *Oh,* no. *Oh,* no. Audrey, we've got a real problem here. If we don't get him help, he's gonna die. Oh, *no, Zoom Zoom!*"

The bottle of Luvox is a few feet away on the ground, the orange plastic under the white cap punctured with teeth marks. Mom must have kept the bottle in her bag of toiletries, which is wide open and tipped over next to her bed.

"Mom, did you look in the bottle? How do you even know he ate some?"

"Because, Audrey, *because!* Look at that *bottle!* He tore into it!"

285

I take my hands off Zoom Zoom and grab it. There's a hole between the cap and top of the teeth marks.

Mom lets go of Zoom Zoom's jaws but wraps her forearms around his neck to keep him put.

"Mom, there are still a lot of pills left!"

"How many?"

I twist off the cap, pour them in my hand, and count.

"Twenty-two pills. There were 30 to begin with. I've had... a total of four. That's 26 that should be left. So that means Zoom Zoom only ate four of them. Mom, he's gonna be fine!"

Her panicked expression says she doesn't believe me.

"Only four pills, Mom. He's not gonna die."

"Okay. Okay. Four pills. Are you *sure* he's only had four?"

"Yes, Mom. I did the math."

"You're sure there were just 30 to begin with?"

"Yes. The bottle doesn't even have room for more than that."

"Okay, you think he had four?"

"Yes. Four."

"Okay. Okay. I gotta call Poison Control. This is not good,

Audrey. Not good."

"Oh my word."

Mom lets go of Zoom Zoom, gets up, and finds a phonebook in the drawer between the beds. I get back into bed, face the wall by the bathroom, and smooth the covers over me. There won't be silence anytime soon, but perhaps I can lie here without Mom forcing me to get back up.

"Audrey, I need help here. I gotta find the number for Poison Control."

I turn my head towards Mom, who is flipping through the phonebook.

"Mom, there's only one phonebook, and Zoom Zoom is fine! I need to be alone! I need some time to myself!"

Her eyeballs are scanning the yellow pages.

"Okay. Okay, here. Here it is. Poison control... Okay, I'm dialing them up... Oh, yes, Zoom Zoom, you are a good boy, and Mommy loves you... Yes, *yes* Mam, you can help me! My dog Zoom Zoom ate some Luvox. That's Fluvoxamine. It's used to treat OCD. My daughter says she thinks he had four pills... Luvox is a serotonin reuptake inhibitor. We are hundreds of miles from home at a hotel... Yes, yes... Okay... You think so? I just don't know where I'd take him... So we need to know how to make sure he's gonna be okay... Okay..."

I can't believe this is my life.

"Okay, yes, please make sure to tell me if he needs to be taken somewhere. We just don't want to take any chances with our sweet Zoom Zoom... You know, Zoom Zoom is one of our strays, and we think he's mentally challenged."

If Mom is taking Zoom Zoom to the vet, I am absolutely not going with her. Mom has done so much for me... but I cannot endure a trip to a vet, not to mention more time in that winnebaga.

"So, it wasn't a significant amount of Luvox?... Oh, I'd say Zoom Zoom weighs about 95 pounds or so. He is tall and lanky."

Whew. He's not going to the vet.

"Okay, Mam, if you're sure then we won't take him. This is a real relief for us. We are so far from home and don't know where we could go or how many hundreds of miles it might take to get there... Okay, thank you so much. That's what we will do."

Mom hangs up the phone and holds out her arms. "Oh, Zoom Zoom, come here!"

"What did she say, Mom?"

"She said she thinks he'll be okay, but he'll need to drink a lot of water... Quick, Zoom Zoom, let's get you some water, boy. You're gonna drink, drink, drink. I'm gonna hafta take you potty all night long and make you keep drinking... That's the only way we can detox you. Good boy, Zoom Zoom. But don't you *ever* do that again!"

Zoom Zoom trots behind Mom to the bathroom sink.

Early September 2009 Brodville, Wisconsin

We got here in four days instead of five. How we did that, with all the stops, is a mystery. We're pulling into the driveway of the 16-acre farm Mom and Todd bought, and four of these acres are fenced-in. Our new house is on the left, a humongous barn is at the end of the driveway, and large trees shade the spacious yard and make me imagine that the grass will feel cool underfoot.

Grass.

I had no sleep on the trip. My body is agitated from sitting for hours, and arriving at our destination has brought me no closer to healing.

That horizon through the front winnebaga window *lied* to me... it suggested something better was ahead.

Todd stops the winnebaga in front of the barn.

I start to cry and run out of the side door. I'm walking barefoot through a grassy field to the right of the barn. I cannot move fast enough to shake off the restlessness of sitting for four days.

"Audrey!" Mom calls, and she tries to come after me.

But I'm walking away fast. "Leave me alone!"

My feet sink into the soft grass and dirt underneath. I'm around the barn and on the other side of the property beyond the house. There are many trees on this side, and breezes are filtering through them. White and gray clouds are gliding above. The sun is behind them and lowering.

Clouds. We are back in the Midwest.

I feel no relief at all. But if I could, it would be in knowing that the California desert is far, far away.

12 And it's not yet Christmas

October 2009 Brodville, Wisconsin

There's a huge field behind our property, a highway in front, and woods on either side.

Mom had this fence put in before we arrived. That way, the dogs would have no chance of running out to the highway and getting hit. Todd hung his tools in the front of the barn when we got here. In the middle of the barn are Todd's two four-wheelers and a scooter, and in the back is his Mustang.

The winnebaga sits outside the barn to the left, never letting me forget the four days on the road within its walls.

Unpacking was the bane of my first two weeks here. Mom insisted I unwrap china, take boxes to the downstairs storage room, and wash the vegetables from the garden left over from the people Mom and Todd bought the farm from. My crying and protesting did nothing to deter her from giving me orders. So I yelled outside on the front lawn one day. I knew what Mom was thinking—that she was going to age ten more years within weeks. I told her she was welcome to send me to an institution. She said nothing.

When Todd got home in the evenings, he put me to work outside, knowing I preferred to be outdoors and needed the distraction of working. When hanging tools or helping wire fence, I looked at the sunset as if God lived behind it. I asked Him to let me die, somehow.

I sensed He understood. I also sensed His answer wasn't yes.

At that time, I didn't imagine I'd soon be getting some sleep.

In those August and September days, I walked the grassy property barefoot and then read recovery stories online for many hours at a time. Some of the stories I read had started out just like mine and concluded with a happy ending, so those meant the most.

The October air is nice and cool, though I am nervous that snow could come as early as this month. I won't know what to do with myself when the property is blanketed with something too cold to step foot in.

Mom and I go to the store frequently and watch movies at night, and these are two of my better distractions. Every evening when Todd gets home, he and Mom unwind with a beer on the front lawn before we eat dinner inside. Then, Todd and Mom and I play scrabble. We played once, and it proved to be as good a distraction as going to the store or watching a movie. So now, we play every single night, and they are doing it just for me. Todd is really good at Scrabble, and Mom and I are naturals with words, so the competition is thick.

Before Todd retires to bed, I ask him if he still thinks I will get better, and he says, "Yes, Augrit. One day at a time. Just one day at a time."

He's right. I only need to get through one day at a time.

The days have become strings of many days, and time keeps passing. A couple weeks ago, I got two hours of sleep near the beginning of the night. I woke up from a deep sleep much like the first 30 minutes I got after getting off Klonopin. Two full hours of it felt amazing. I immediately pined for more, but also reveled in the taste of normalcy. I recorded the two hours on a calendar the next morning and then recorded my sleep each morning after. Since then I have gotten two and sometimes three hours of sleep most nights.

I can remember what it's like to sleep now. I also feel almost okay at more moments of the day. The people on the benzo forums call these times "windows"—short periods of feeling normal again. They say the windows get longer and more frequent.

Now that I've got windows, my despair has lessened. I have stopped asking God for permission to die. I have begun to believe I will heal someday. It could be one year or it could be three. But, I think I will heal. There's only one way to find out for sure—and that is by staying alive.

293

I discovered a place to walk other than the land inside our fence. Mom said if I go out the metal gate, there is a country road immediately to the right. I walk it every day for a couple of miles. It is lined with woods and then little farms with houses and barns. The woods keep the sun at bay and allow for breezes. Sometimes I venture down other side roads.

My heart is more open on these walks, perhaps because a little sleep has come back. I look ahead on the country road as far as I can see, and I think of my destination—the only one I'm sure of. I don't know what my life will become, but, at the end, I believe I will meet Jesus. A priest said to me once that this life is just the introduction. I may not have a family of my own, nearby friends, a job, or even the ability to sleep much, but what I have is worth more than the whole world: I believe Jesus will raise me from the dead and let me be with Him forever.

I have *hope*. One way I know that is I am journaling again. Mom has me in a pretty light-green painted room with an Indian-print blanket. There is a bedside wood table and a lamp—but not the parrot lamp; that sits in the dining room. After Mom says goodnight and shuts the door, I write. The other night my heart was not only open but very warm. God must have done that—the inside of me was like a bath bubbling up. I felt loved and embraced, and I perceived a Being Who is good—very good. I wrote:

"I don't know my future. I don't even know for sure if I will heal from this condition or what my life will be. But I know that my life matters. God has a plan for my life, and His plan is good."

No matter what happens, His plan is to do something good with it all. I didn't believe this before, but I sense it now.

It's the second week of October, and for the very first time in months, I felt normal all day long.

I think that I might be alright someday.

Last night I slept for seven hours. *Seven hours?* It doesn't seem real. I did what I thought I couldn't do, and without trying. Some of the sleep was light. I certainly woke up a lot. But today I feel normal... my longest "window" so far.

Normal.

Mom let me take the car out. I went grocery shopping and got everything on her list. I relished the sights and scents. When I got home, I washed dishes and looked out the window at the lowering sun, seeing the breeze bend the grass on the property and hearing the chimes on the front porch. Mom loves chimes. The breeze was a lot like the one on The Back Nine—it whirled around a beautiful piece of property and made me sense that the One behind it is good.

It's evening now, and I don't know what tonight will bring. It could be another good night, or it could be a wide-awake one. But it doesn't matter because I am living in the moment right now—it's easy to.

I'm feeling better, and it's not yet Christmas.

AFTERWORD

That first good night's sleep in mid-October was the longest "window" I'd had. The next day, the window shut, and I experienced sleeplessness for many days just as I had in the beginning of withdrawal. Members on the forum often said they felt as bad as ever following a good window. I took that to heart, hoping I was getting better.

The third week of October, I was invited to live with extended family in Indiana. One day, in the middle of November, I noticed that my mood was positive and that I'd gotten a significant amount of sleep the night before. I had an inkling that, just perhaps, my time of healing had come.

Within a week, which was the week before Thanksgiving, all my natural sleep returned. I felt as if someone had let me out of a prison. My life began again, and I couldn't wait to live it. I had read that benzo withdrawal often lasts six months or longer, and mine had lasted only five and a half months. I certainly had not anticipated such a positive turn-a-round so quickly. For some time, however, I struggled to believe that I really had healed. I even feared that my brain was still damaged, although I functioned and slept well. Only after I recovered did I have 100% certainty that I had suffered from benzo withdrawal; up to that point, there had been no way for me to entirely give up the paranoia that there was something else wrong with me.

At the time my sleep came back, I made the fortunate discovery of sleep trackers and purchased one. Because my sleep tracker assured me I was sleeping, it greatly helped me ward off my tormenting fear of insomnia. After enduring many wide-awake-staring-at-the-clock nights, it was difficult for me to recognize REM sleep and light sleep when they came back; I had many thoughts and even dreams of being awake while in light sleep and REM sleep. The sleep tracker recognized these stages of sleep I had started to get and also helped me turn my brain off when I went to bed. For these reasons, the sleep tracker was indispensable during my recovery.

November 2014 will mark five years since recovering from withdrawal, and in this time I have slept well. I have experienced nothing resembling those five and a half months in withdrawal. I sleep better now than I ever have in my adult years, and I believe this is due to adding more nutrients to my diet.

My experience was with Klonopin, but my book may resonate with experiences of withdrawal from other benzodiazepines and from sleeping pills that are not benzos. I have read that some people have withdrawn from benzodiazepines and sleeping pills with little or no trouble and that some have suffered far more withdrawal symptoms and for a longer period of time than I did. Since insomnia was my primary withdrawal symptom, my heart especially goes out to people who have or are struggling with this issue. I hope my story has encouraged them in particular and shown that things can get better even when it seems otherwise. If my story has helped even one person, then writing this book has been worth it.

RESOURCES

When I was in withdrawal, I did not feel helped by nutritious raw food, supplements, colon cleansing, or anything else. However, when I recovered, I found that what I ate made a huge difference in how I felt and slept. Though I did not personally experience a cure for benzo withdrawal other than time, I do believe that being as healthy as possible enabled me to feel good when that time of recovery came.

Resources for general health that have benefitted me and are available online are The Weston A. Price Foundation, Chris Beat Cancer, and The World's Healthiest Foods. I also recommend the books *Green for Life* by Victoria Boutenko and *Oil Pulling Therapy* by Bruce Fife.

Other than an occasional ibuprofen for aches or pains, I don't take any drugs. I sleep in a dark room with earplugs, a noise machine, and a comfortable temperature. I dim the lighting and try to avoid electronics at least an hour before bed (but two hours is much better). I avoid caffeine twelve hours before bed and rarely drink alcohol. I don't spend more time in bed than I'm able to sleep. I journal and pray when something is bothering me. I have found being at peace to be very important for my sleep quality.

To get the best possible night's sleep, I rely on sunlight, exercise, and, most importantly, nutrients from nutrient-dense foods and food-derived vitamins and minerals.

Klonopin Withdrawal & Howling Dogs: Maybe it was God
is self-published. You'll find it on CreateSpace.com and
Amazon.com. If you believe my book may benefit someone,
please share. Thank you! -Audrey

Made in the USA
Lexington, KY
13 October 2014